T0264070

Complications in Cosmetic Facial Surgery

Guest Editor

JOSEPH NIAMTU III, DMD

ORAL AND MAXILLOFACIAL SURGERY CLINICS OF NORTH AMERICA

www.oralmaxsurgery.theclinics.com

Consulting Editor
RICHARD H. HAUG, DDS

February 2009 • Volume 21 • Number 1

SAUNDERS an imprint of ELSEVIER, Inc.

W.B. SAUNDERS COMPANY
A Division of Elsevier Inc.

1600 John F. Kennedy Blvd. ● Suite 1800 ● Philadelphia, PA 19103-2899

http://www.theclinics.com

ORAL AND MAXILLOFACIAL SURGERY CLINICS OF NORTH AMERICA Volume 21, Number 1
February 2009 ISSN 1042-3699, ISBN-13: 978-1-4377-0512-6, ISBN-10: 1-4377-0512-X

Editor: John Vassallo; j.vassallo@elsevier.com
Developmental Editor: Donald Mumford

© **2009 Elsevier** ■ **All rights reserved.**

This journal and the individual contributions contained in it are protected under copyright by Elsevier, and the following terms and conditions apply to their use:

Photocopying
Single photocopies of single articles may be made for personal use as allowed by national copyright laws. Permission of the Publisher and payment of a fee is required for all other photocopying, including multiple or systematic copying, copying for advertising or promotional purposes, resale, and all forms of document delivery. Special rates are available for educational institutions that wish to make photocopies for non-profit educational classroom use.
For information on how to seek permission visit www.elsevier.com/permissions or call: (+44) 1865 843830 (UK)/(+1) 215 239 3804 (USA).

Derivative Works
Subscribers may reproduce tables of contents or prepare lists of articles including abstracts for internal circulation within their institutions. Permission of the Publisher is required for resale or distribution outside the institution. Permission of the Publisher is required for all other derivative works, including compilations and translations (please consult www.elsevier.com/permissions).

Electronic Storage or Usage
Permission of the Publisher is required to store or use electronically any material contained in this journal, including any article or part of an article (please consult www.elsevier.com/permissions). Except as outlined above, no part of this publication may be reproduced, stored in a retrieval system or transmitted in any form or by any means, electronic, mechanical, photocopying, recording or otherwise, without prior written permission of the Publisher.

Notice
No responsibility is assumed by the Publisher for any injury and/or damage to persons or property as a matter of products liability, negligence or otherwise, or from any use or operation of any methods, products, instructions or ideas contained in the material herein. Because of rapid advances in the medical sciences, in particular, independent verification of diagnoses and drug dosages should be made.

Although all advertising material is expected to conform to ethical (medical) standards, inclusion in this publication does not constitute a guarantee or endorsement of the quality or value of such product or of the claims made of it by its manufacturer.

Oral and Maxillofacial Surgery Clinics of North America (ISSN 1042-3699) is published quarterly by Elsevier Inc., 360 Park Avenue South, New York, NY 10010-1710. Months of issue are February, May, August, and November. Business and Editorial Offices: 1600 John F. Kennedy Blvd., Suite 1800, Philadelphia, PA 19103-2899. Periodicals postage paid at New York, NY and additional mailing offices. Subscription prices are $271.00 per year for US individuals, $401.00 per year for US institutions, $125.00 per year for US students and residents, $313.00 per year for Canadian individuals, $478.00 per year for Canadian institutions, $362.00 per year for international individuals, $478.00 per year for international institutions and $170.00 per year for Canadian and foreign students/residents. To receive student/resident rate, orders must be accompanied by name or affiliated institution, date of term, and the *signature* of program/residency coordinator on institution letterhead. Orders will be billed at individual rate until proof of status is received. Foreign air speed delivery is included in all *Clinics* subscription prices. All prices are subject to change without notice. **POSTMASTER:** Send address changes to *Oral and Maxillofacial Surgery Clinics of North America,* Elsevier Periodicals Customer Service, 11830 Westline Industrial Drive, St. Louis, MO 63146. Tel: 1-800-654-2452 (U.S. and Canada); 314-453-7041 (outside U.S. and Canada). Fax: 314-523-5170. E-mail: journalscustomerservice-usa@elsevier.com (for print support); journalsonlinesupport-usa@elsevier.com (for online support).

Reprints. For copies of 100 or more, of articles in this publication, please contact the Commercial Reprints Department, Elsevier Inc., 360 Park Avenue South, New York, NY 10010-1710. Tel.: 212-633-3812; Fax: 212-462-1935; Email: reprints@elsevier.com.

Oral and Maxillofacial Surgery Clinics of North America is covered in MEDLINE/PubMed (*Index Medicus*).

Printed and bound by CPI Group (UK) Ltd, Croydon, CR0 4YY

Transferred to Digital Print 2011

Contributors

GUEST EDITOR

JOSEPH NIAMTU III, DMD
Cosmetic Facial Surgery, Richmond, Virginia

AUTHORS

BABAK AZIZZADEH, MD, FACS
Assistant Clinical Professor, Division of
Head & Neck Surgery, David Geffen School
of Medicine at UCLA, Los Angeles, California

TERESA G. BIGGERSTAFF, DDS, MD
Fellow, Carolina Surgical Arts, Greensboro,
North Carolina

GERALD C. CANAAN II, JD
Director, Hancock, Daniel, Johnson & Nagle,
Glen Allen, Virginia

L. ANGELO CUZALINA, MD, DDS
Co-director, American Academy of Cosmetic
Surgery Fellowship, Tulsa Surgical Arts, Tulsa,
Oklahoma

MARK J. GLASGOLD, MD, FACS
Clinical Associate Professor, Department
of Surgery, University of Medicine & Dentistry
of New Jersey, Robert Wood Johnson Medical
School, Piscataway; and Glasgold Group
Plastic Surgery, Highland Park, New Jersey

ROBERT A. GLASGOLD, MD
Clinical Assistant Professor, Department
of Surgery, University of Medicine & Dentistry
of New Jersey, Robert Wood Johnson Medical
School, Piscataway; and Glasgold Group
Plastic Surgery, Highland Park, New Jersey

BRIAN C. HARSHA, DDS, MS
Private Practice, Coastal Facial Aesthetic &
Laser Surgery, Myrtle Beach, South Carolina

MORRIS E. HARTSTEIN, MD, FACS
Clinical Associate Professor of Ophthalmology,
Saint Louis University Eye Institute, Saint Louis
University School of Medicine, St. Louis,
Missouri

MATTHEW R. HLAVACEK, MD, DDS
Fellow, American Academy of Cosmetic
Surgery Fellowship, Tulsa Surgical Arts, Tulsa,
Oklahoma

W. SCOTT JOHNSON, JD
Director, Hancock, Daniel, Johnson & Nagle,
Glen Allen, Virginia

DON KIKKAWA, MD
Professor of Ophthalmology, Shiley Eye
Center, University of California, San Diego,
California

JAMES KOEHLER, MD, DDS
Private Practice; and Co-director, American
Academy Cosmetic Surgery Fellowship, Tulsa
Surgical Arts, Tulsa, Oklahoma

SAMUEL M. LAM, MD, FACS
Director, Willow Bend Wellness Center,
Lam Facial Plastic Surgery Center & Hair
Restoration Institute, Plano, Texas

GRIGORIY MASHKEVICH, MD
Assistant Professor, Division of Facial Plastic
Surgery, Department of Otolaryngology, New
York Eye & Ear Infirmary, New York, New York

JOSEPH NIAMTU III, DMD
Cosmetic Facial Surgery, Richmond, Virginia

ROBERT NIEDBALSKI, DO
Medical Hair Restoration, Bellevue, Washington

SUZAN OBAGI, MD
Associate Professor; and Director, UPMC Cosmetic Surgery and Skin Health Center, Department of Dermatology, University of Pittsburgh Medical Center, Sewickley, Pennsylvania

TODD G. OWSLEY, DDS, MD
Director, Cosmetic Surgery Fellowship; and Private Practice, Carolina Surgical Arts, Greensboro, North Carolina

DAVID PEREZ-MEZA, MD
Private Practice (Plastic and Hair Transplant Surgery Center), Mexico City, Mexico

ALEXANDRA Y. ZHANG, MD
Instructor, Department of Dermatology, University of Pittsburgh Medical Center, Pittsburgh, Pennsylvania

Contents

understanding of the goals of blepharoplasty and the areas for potential problems, we hope to reduce the possibility of developing complications.

Patients desiring improved neck and jawline contours often are looking for minimally invasive procedures and are not interested in undergoing extensive face-lifting procedures. Realizing the limitations, surgeons may offer their patient such procedures as liposuction and submentoplasty. Even though these procedures are less involved than a facelift, many pitfalls can occur, leading to an unfavorable result and a disappointed patient. Proper patient selection and choosing the correct operation are crucial to avoiding these situations. This article focuses on the common complications of neck liposuction and submentoplasty and reviews the management and avoidance of these complications.

Traditionally, strategies for facial rejuvenation have emphasized correction of tissue ptosis and laxity with suspensory and excisional techniques, such as face-lifting and blepharoplasty. Volume loss plays a significant role in facial aging and, until recently, had not received appropriate attention. Facial fat grafting to correct volume loss has become a crucial component of facial rejuvenation in the authors' respective practices.

The purpose of this article is to discuss the pros and cons of various aspects of rhytidectomy surgery. The author presents his experiences that have led to performing approximately 85 facelifts a year and what has proved beneficial along the way over the past decade in his cosmetic facial practice. Because it is impossible to incorporate all aspects of facelift complications into the confines of this article, the author focuses on some of the more common problematic and avoidable complications.

Rhinoplasty presents a unique set of challenges for the cosmetic surgeon. Complications may arise from inadequate diagnosis, errors in surgical technique, or variations in the patient's anatomy or healing response. Complications as a result of overly aggressive surgery may also have functional consequences and be harder to correct.

Facial implants are readily used for aesthetic and reconstructive efforts in lieu of autogenous materials due to obvious benefits. Alloplastic facial augmentation is not without potential complications. This article discusses the major factors that contribute to complications of facial implant surgery, based on alloplast composition, surgical technique, and facial region. Also discussed are the most common complications as well as both their prevention and management.

Otoplasty, the correction of protruding ears, is a commonly performed cosmetic surgical procedure. Although few and rare, otoplasty has associated risks and complications. Most of these complications can be minimized by appropriate patient selection, careful preoperative analysis and planning, meticulous surgical technique, and compliant postoperative care. The surgeon must be familiar with the possible complications to avoid or prevent them. The astute surgeon must also be able to recognize and confidently treat adverse outcomes as they occur to minimize long-term sequelae.

Hair loss affects more than 1.2 billion people worldwide. As the technology and artistry of hair restoration surgery has improved including natural results, so too has the popularity of this procedure. As with any other surgical procedure, complications may occur and this presents a major challenge for the surgeon and the patient. This article provides an overview of the complications most likely to occur during the pre, intra, and postoperative periods with modern hair transplant surgery (single follicular unit or multifollicular unit) including scalp surgery, and discusses their treatment and most importantly their prevention.

Oral and maxillofacial surgeons can improve patient relationships by pretending that patients are potential jurors. Looking at relationships from the eyes of a juror allows oral and maxillofacial surgeons to ascertain patients' personality types and modify communication styles accordingly. This approach also allows oral and maxillofacial surgeons to understand why patients (jurors) need to see information and evidence.

Oral and Maxillofacial Surgery Clinics of North America

THE CLINICS ARE NOW AVAILABLE ONLINE!

Access your subscription at:
www.theclinics.com

Preface

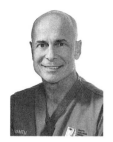

Joseph Niamtu III, DMD
Guest Editor

A revolution is occurring in the field of cosmetic surgery as it has become an accepted, requested, and welcome part of contemporary society. Many changes have happened over the past 40 years. Cosmetic facial surgery has been around in some shape or form for centuries. However, it became a predictable procedure only after advances in anesthesia, surgery, and antibiotics. Forty years ago, cosmetic surgery was a well-kept secret of the rich and famous. People who sought out the procedure then were on average older then those seeking it today, and many of them would sneak away to have the procedure done secretly. The procedures were expensive and extensive, and many produced an unnatural appearance. Much has changed. Baby boomers, now in their sixth decade, don't want to look old and hence are having surgery earlier. They tend to prefer smaller procedures at a younger age to avoid the "overhaul" their parents had. With the increased focus on youth, health, and beauty, cosmetic surgery has worked itself into the fabric of mainstream life and pop culture and has become a rite of passage in aging for many patients.

Along with this phenomenal growth of cosmetic surgery came another paradigm shift: Numerous specialties began providing cosmetic procedures. Although plastic surgery controlled cosmetic surgery in the past, today 80% of cosmetic surgery is performed by non–plastic surgeons. So, now we have had exponential growth of patients with a similar growth of providers. It only made sense that the number of surgery complications would also grow.

Complications are a normal part of surgery. No surgeon is immune. Complications can stem from uncontrollable factors, such as the patient's immune system and healing; from preventable or controllable factors, such as nonsterile surgical environments; or from incompetence or mistakes on the part of the surgeon or staff. Complications can occur in the preoperative, intraoperative, and postoperative phases of cosmetic facial surgery. Someone once said, "Most complications are proximal to the scalpel," which means that they are the fault of the surgeon. It is probably safe to say that the average surgeon has more complications on the upslope of his or her learning curve. Having said this, even the most competent and experienced surgeons experience complications. Although dreaded, complications have much to teach surgeons about preventing them or limiting them in the future. One of the biggest mistakes a surgeon can make is to see a patient from another colleague and "bad-mouth" that colleague's ability or competence. What goes around comes around and surgeons who speak badly of colleagues will most likely be subject of similar remarks some day.

All surgeons can and must learn from complications as well as have a firm understanding of their pathophysiology and how to prevent them. The purpose of this volume is to present the more common complications that accompany cosmetic facial surgery. Surgeons should be forthright about their complications. The profession and public can see right through those surgeons who claim never to have complications. It is my hope that readers will gain valuable information on what causes common complications and on how they can improve their practices and techniques to limit or prevent them. Obviously, a volume of this size cannot discuss the entire scope of all complications, so we have focused on the "garden variety" commonly seen in the cosmetic facial surgery practice. Because some aspects of

Oral Maxillofacial Surg Clin N Am 21 (2009) ix–x
doi:10.1016/j.coms.2008.11.003
1042-3699/08/$ – see front matter © 2009 Elsevier Inc. All rights reserved.

oralmaxsurgery.theclinics.com

complications are subjective, it is not uncommon for different practitioners to have different ideas about the cause and prevention of complications.

The process of dealing with complications begins before they occur—at the preoperative stage. Because most complications are predictable (for example, 2% of facelift patients will have a hematoma), the informed consent and patient process should include a discussion of the common (and uncommon) complications. It has been said that when a problem is discussed preoperatively it is a sequela, but when it is discussed postoperatively it is a complication. Very true. We owe it to our patients to inform them of the possible complications that accompany their proposed surgery. Surgeons who fail to obtain written consents are difficult to defend in the courtroom. Lawsuits are an unsavory part of cosmetic surgery for both the patient and the surgeon. No one wants complications to happen and every good surgeon takes them and their impact on the patient seriously. A complication on a cardiac patient during efforts to save that patient's life may go unchallenged, but, with elective cosmetic procedures (cosmetic surgery is never required), a patient who came in to look better and now looks worse is definitely more likely to pursue legal options. The late Julius Newman, a cosmetic surgery pioneer, was correct when he said, "If you do this type of work, expect problems."

I am truly honored to have had the opportunity to assemble contributors who are among the leaders in their specialties in cosmetic facial surgery. The breadth of their knowledge and experience make this a truly valuable volume for any practitioner in any specialty that performs cosmetic facial surgery.

It is my hope that this volume will serve both as a guide for managing complications and as a preventive primer for avoiding them.

Joseph Niamtu III, DMD
11319 Polo Place
Midlothian, VA 23113, USA

E-mail address:
niamtu@niamtu.com

Diagnosis and Management of Skin Resurfacing–Related Complications

Alexandra Y. Zhang, MD[a], Suzan Obagi, MD[b],*

KEYWORDS

- Chemical peel • Laser resurfacing • Dermabrasion • Laser
- Broadband light • Infection • Scar • Skin conditioning

Skin resurfacing, especially minimally invasive skin resurfacing, has gained increasing popularity among physicians and patients because of its rapid recovery, low risks for complications, and gratifying results. Skin resurfacing is a field of rapid evolution, with many new technologies that have developed over the years, and has been used extensively by physicians in a variety of specialties to achieve cosmetic enhancement. Thorough understanding of the anatomy and pathophysiology of skin, proper patient evaluation, appropriate selection of procedures based on different skin types, and underscoring potential complications of each procedure, however, are essential to achieve optimal results and to minimize complications related to skin resurfacing.

Skin serves as a physiologic barrier to prevent fluid loss and to protect the human body from exposure to trauma, ultraviolet radiation, infections, and toxins. Other major functions of the skin include sensory perception, immune recognition, and thermoregulation. The skin is composed of two layers, epidermis and dermis, that overlie the subcutaneous fat (Fig. 1). The epidermis is approximately 50 μm in thickness and consists of three major resident cells: keratinocytes, Langerhans' cells, and melanocytes. The melanocytes are capable of producing and transferring melanin. The dermis contains vascular structures and nerves endings in a collagen- and elastin-containing matrix, which provides circulation and nutritional and structural support for the epidermis (see Fig. 1). Fibroblasts, macrophages, and dendritic cells are the main resident cells in the dermis. Fibroblasts produce the collagen, elastin, and glycosaminoglycans that constitute the dermal matrix. Epidermal adnexal structures include eccrine glands, apocrine glands, sebaceous glands, and hair follicles. It is these adnexal structures that play an important role in skin reepithelialization when the overlying epidermis is removed by traumatic abrasions, dermabrasion, chemical peeling, or ablative laser skin resurfacing.

COMMON COMPLICATIONS FROM MOST TYPES OF SKIN RESURFACING MODALITIES

Skin resurfacing is accomplished by controlled skin injury to remodel the epidermis or dermis, results in smoothing of surface irregularities, and stimulates new collagen synthesis to achieve an enhanced cosmetic appearance. Many modalities have been used for resurfacing, such as chemical peels, photodynamic therapy (PDT), microdermabrasion, dermabrasion, ablative and nonablative lasers, and fractional lasers. Most resurfacing-related complications are associated with the depth of the wound created rather than the type of modality used. To achieve tightening of the skin, the depth of the wound must approach

[a] Department of Dermatology, University of Pittsburgh Medical Center, Pittsburgh, PA, USA
[b] Cosmetic Surgery and Skin Health Center, Department of Dermatology, University of Pittsburgh Medical Center, 1603 Carmody Court, Suite 103, Blaymore Building II, Sewickley, PA 15143, USA
* Corresponding author.
E-mail address: obagimd@gmail.com (S. Obagi).

Oral Maxillofacial Surg Clin N Am 21 (2009) 1–12
doi:10.1016/j.coms.2008.11.002
1042-3699/08/$ – see front matter © 2009 Elsevier Inc. All rights reserved.

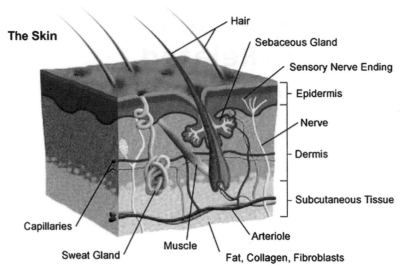

The Skin

Hair
Sebaceous Gland
Sensory Nerve Ending
Epidermis
Nerve
Dermis
Subcutaneous Tissue
Capillaries
Arteriole
Muscle
Sweat Gland
Fat, Collagen, Fibroblasts

Fig. 1. Skin anatomy diagram showing the epidermis, dermis, and subcutaneous fat. Note that many of the adnexal structures are located in the dermis.

the papillary dermis. To achieve leveling of the skin surface, however, the wound depth must approach the upper reticular dermis. Thus, skin laxity is addressed with tightening levels of skin resurfacing, whereas certain acne scars and deeper rhytides require a leveling depth of wounding. As the depth of wounding exceeds the upper reticular dermis, however, the risks for permanent pigmentary changes, textual changes, and scarring increase significantly. It is essential, therefore, to control the depth of the wounding to obtain the maximal desired clinical effects with minimal complications. Other complications of resurfacing include contact dermatitis, milia formation, infection, acne and rosacea flares, postinflammatory pigmentary changes, prolonged erythema, and so forth (**Box 1**).

Acute complications occur within the first few days up to 1 month after the procedure. Long-term complications become apparent after the initial 2 weeks of healing from skin resurfacing.

Contact Dermatitis

Contact dermatitis, usually irritant in nature, is seen commonly after skin resurfacing as a result of impaired epidermal barrier function.[1–3] It rarely is a true type IV delayed hypersensitivity reaction because patch testing fails to reveal the allergens in most cases. Patients usually complain of burning and itching sensation of their skin along with increased redness. Eczematous eruptions also may occur (**Fig. 2**). Contact dermatitis may occur during the first 4 weeks after resurfacing. The deepithelialized state of the skin after resurfacing renders increased susceptibility to topical irritants,

such as fragrances, propylene glycol, or lanolin and allergens in cleansers, moisturizes, and topical ointments, during the reepithelialization process. It is important to have patients avoid self-prescribed, topical, so-called herbal regimens or topical antibiotics, such as Neosporin (Johnson & Johnson) or bacitracin during the healing process. Once patients present with symptoms of contact dermatitis, immediate discontinuation of probable offending agents, cool compresses,

---

Box 1
Acute and long-term complications associated with skin resurfacing procedures

Acute complications

Contact dermatitis

Bacteria, fungal, and viral infections

Erythema

Pseudohypopigmentation

Delayed wound healing

Transient postinflammatory hyper- or hypopigmentation

Acne and rosacea flare

Milia

Long-term complications

Prolonged erythema

Pigmentary changes

Textural changes

Scarring (hypertrophic and atrophic)

Keloid formation

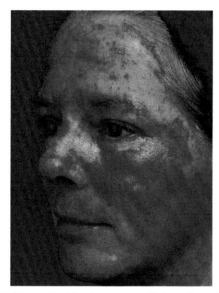

Fig. 2. The patient had an uneventful medium-depth peel that was complicated on postoperative day 4 by healing regression and pruritus. This was caused by propylene glycol in one of her postoperative products.

application of mid-potency topical steroids, and administration of oral antihistamines are helpful to alleviate pruritus and cutaneous eruptions. In severe cases, the use of ultrapotent topical steroids is indicated. The use of steroids should be monitored closely, however, to avoid steroid-induced delayed wound healing.

Bacterial, Fungal, and Viral Infections

Rapid onset of pain and swelling and focal areas of increased erythema, purulence, malodorous discharge, erosions, and crusting are signs of bacterial infection (**Fig. 3**A). *Staphylococcus aureus* and *Pseudomonas aeruginosa* are the species isolated most commonly.[4] Wound culture should be performed if an infection is suspected to identify the organism and to obtain drug sensitivities. Bacterial infections often develop between postoperative days 2 and 10. *Staphylococcus aureus* is the most common cause in open wounds. If a wound is occluded for more than 48 hours, however, or if prophylactic antibiotics are used, the incidence of a gram-negative infection, including *Pseudomonas aeruginosa*, is increased significantly. Occlusive dressings create a moist environment over necrotic tissue, creating a perfect medium for the growth of various organisms that contributes to increased incidence of postresurfacing bacterial infections.[4] Therefore, meticulous wound care with decreased duration of occlusion, frequent dressing changes, and thorough cleaning of wounds with 0.25% acetic acid solution are effective in reducing bacterial colonization. The routine use of prophylactic antibiotics is controversial although it is recommended for patients who have increased risks for infections. A study conducted by Walia and Alster[5,6] did not show decreased rate of cutaneous infection in 133 patients undergoing full-face CO_2 laser resurfacing when prophylactic antibiotics were used. If a bacterial infection is suspected, however, broad-spectrum systemic antibiotics, such as penicillins, cephalosporins, or ciprofloxacin, should be given to patients while waiting for the results of bacterial culture with antibiotic sensitivities.

Candida albicans is the most common fungal/yeast species causing wound infections after skin resurfacing that occur at approximately postoperative day 5. Usually patients are healing well

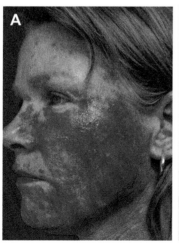
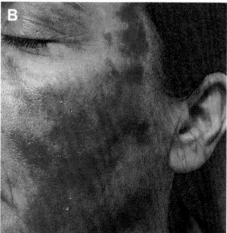

Fig. 3. (*A*) A patient who had *Staphylococcal aureus* infection on postoperative day 4 after a medium-depth peel. This patient presented with slightly increase swelling and new onset of pain. (*B*) Patient who had painful erosions on the skin without the classic vesicles seen in HSV.

until a *Candida* infection sets in. At this point, wound healing begins to regress and patients begin to develop symptoms ranging from pruritus to painful erosions.[7] Potassium hydroxide slide preparation should be performed if *Candida* infection is suspected. Wound care with frequent dressing changes and cleaning wounds with diluted acetic acid, topical antiyeast cream, silver sulfadiazene cream, or oral fluconozole can be used in the treatment of postoperative fungal infection.[6,7]

Reactivation of herpes simplex virus (HSV) after skin resurfacing can be disastrous. It is critical to recognize and treat infections to prevent delayed wound healing, disseminated viral infection, secondary infections with opportunistic pathogens, and scarring. Because the skin is deepithelialized, postresurfacing herpetic infection may present only as superficial erosions but not as classic vesiculopustules that appear on normal skin (**Fig. 4**). Other associated symptoms, such as pruritus or dysthesia, may accompany delayed wound healing. Because many HSV infections can be subclinical, patients who plan to undergo full-face or perioral resurfacing should receive oral antiviral prophylaxis, such as acyclovir, famciclovir, or valacyclovir. The prophylaxis should be initiated 1 to 2 days before the resurfacing and continued for 7 days (medium-depth peels and light laser resurfacing) to 15 days (dermabrasion, traditional laser resurfacing, and deep peels) until reepithelialization of the skin is complete.[8] Despite appropriate prophylactic antiviral therapy, however, some patients experience an outbreak only while on a suppressive regimen.[2,9] If a HSV infection is suspected, aggressive antiviral therapy should be administered at an equivalent dose to treat herpes zoster. In situations of disseminated herpes infection, intravenous administration of antiviral therapy with hospital admission is warranted.

Other unusual infections also may occur after skin resurfacing. Rao and colleagues[10] reported a case of atypical mycobacterial infection with *Mycobacterium fortuitum* after full-face skin resurfacing with CO_2 laser that presented as nontender, erythematous nodules. The nodules resolved after multiple incisions and drainage and a 4-week course of oral ciprofloxacin. Usually mycobacterial infection presents 4 to 6 weeks out from surgery. This often is missed on routine tissue culture unless specified on the request slip. Although atypical mycobacterial infection is a rare complication of skin resurfacing, it is important to keep it in the differential diagnosis when patients do not respond to traditional wound care, antibiotics, or antifungal or antiviral therapies and if patients present with a late-onset infection.

Milia

Milia usually develop between 3 and 8 weeks after ablative skin resurfacing and often are related to the depth of wounding. These keratin-retention cysts may be isolated or in clusters and can be disturbing to patients. Milia formation is caused by plugged hair follicles secondary to the use of occlusive dressings or ointments during the wound healing process. In most cases, milia resolve spontaneously as the skin continues to reepithelialize or with just regular postoperative cleansing. Topical application of retinoic acid, glycolic acid therapy, and manual extraction also are helpful modalities to facilitate the resolution of milia.[11–13]

Acne and Rosacea Flare

Postoperative acne and rosacea flares are common and can occur in as many as 80% of patients who undergo laser resurfacing (see **Fig. 4**).[1–3] Patients whose acne and rosacea are not well controlled before skin resurfacing are more prone to having flares after the procedure. Proper topical regimens in combination with oral antibiotics, such as tetracycline, doxycycline, and minocycline, should be used before scarring ensues.

Prolonged Erythema

Postoperative erythema is an expected consequence of skin resurfacing.[2,3] Prolonged erythema (>3 weeks postoperatively) can be a challenging complication. When it lasts for more than 3 months, it can be frustrating for patients and

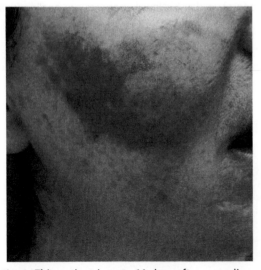

Fig. 4. This patient is seen 14 days after a medium-depth peel with erythema and papules on the cheeks consistent with a rosacea flare.

physicians. Although prolonged erythema can occur with any skin resurfacing modality, it seems to occur more often with ablative laser resurfacing than with dermabrasion and chemical peels.[14] It is more likely to occur in areas with delayed wound healing or in areas resurfaced to the level of the reticular dermis. The exact mechanism of prolonged erythema is uncertain but may be associated with resurfacing-induced inflammatory response, reduced absorption of light by melanin, and decreased optical scattering in the dermis.[15] Several factors have been identified as contributing to increased risks for postoperative prolonged erythema, such as multiple passes or overlapping passes during ablative laser resurfacing, aggressive intraoperative débridement of desiccated skin tissue, postoperative contact dermatitis, and delayed would healing secondary to infection, trauma, or irritation.

Any topical regimen used with the intention of treating postoperative erythema before the completion of reepithelialization process may irritate the denuded skin and worsen the erythema. Topical application of ascorbic acid after reepithelialization of the skin has been shown to reduce the duration and severity of erythema. The role of topical corticosteroids in the treatment of postoperative erythema is controversial. Some studies indicate that postoperative use of topical corticosteroids seemed to be a cause of prolonged erythema and telangiectasias because of the effects of vasoconstriction and vasodilatation through a nonintact barrier.[16] Focal areas of prolonged erythema, however, with tenderness could be signs of scarring (**Fig. 5**A, B); therefore, topical application of ultrapotent class I steroids to the area 2 days a week for several weeks can be used to prevent scar formation. Close patient monitoring is necessary to avoid adverse effects. Flashlamp pulsed dye laser or other low-level laser treatment also is an effective modality in cases of recalcitrant prolonged erythema. Subpurpuric doses with more frequent treatments (every 1 to 2 weeks) can be used until the erythema subsides.

Pigmentary Alteration

Any wounding of the skin, superficial or deep, can trigger a hyperpigmentation response in susceptible patients. The severity and longevity of this usually correlate with wound depth. Pigment alteration after skin resurfacing can be transient or long term. Transient postinflammatory hyperpigmentation (PIH) is one of the most common complications associated with resurfacing. It can occur in approximately one third of patients postoperatively regardless of skin type.[2,3,17] In white patients, those who have darker skin tones (brunettes) are more at risk for PIH. In Asian skin or black skin, however, patients who have lighter skin tones are more prone to PIH.[18] These patients usually present with freckling, melasma, or other dyschromia at baseline. Additionally, patients who have a suntan have a much higher risk for developing PIH that can last for several months if left untreated[19] as their melanocytes already are stimulated. Although most hyperpigmentation is transient, it usually is noticeable and the majority of patients seek treatment to speed up its resolution (**Fig. 6**A, B). The regular use of broad-spectrum sunscreens for at least 6 to 8 weeks before the resurfacing procedure and postoperatively are critical to prevent ultraviolet light-induced melanin synthesis and thus achieve and maintain the optimal result of resurfacing. Topical bleaching agents, such as hydroquinone, kojic acid, retinoic acid, azelaic acid, ascorbic acid, glycolic acid, and physical sunblock, are first-line treatments for PIH. In recalcitrant cases, superficial light chemical peels with glycolic acid (30% to 40%) and salicylic

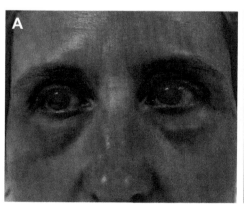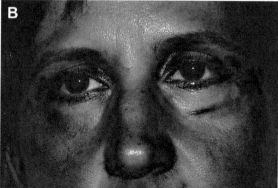

Fig. 5. (*A*) Prolonged erythema seen here at postoperative day 22, which has progressed to a hypertrophic scar seen here at 3 months (*B*) after a chemical peel.

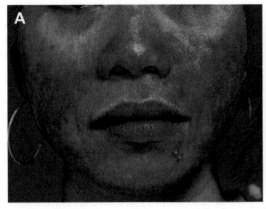
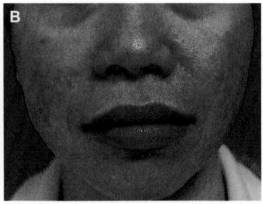

Fig. 6. Transient PIH in an Asian patient (*A*) after a pulsed dye laser and a medium-depth chemical peel. This resolved with topical agents and weekly salicylic acid peels (*B*) as seen 3 months postoperatively.

acid (30%) or microdermabrasion (biweekly, may repeat every 2 to 4 weeks as needed) can hasten the resolution of hyperpigmentation.[17,20] Improper topical treatment before reepitheliazation of the skin should be avoided, however, because it can aggravate the severity of PIH. The proper use of a skin-conditioning program before and after resurfacing greatly reduces the risk for PIH. The duration of the preconditioning program is adjusted to patients' skin type and risk for PIH.[21] Therefore, patients deemed at risk for PIH should be preconditioned for 3 months rather than the standard 6 weeks. Likewise, the duration of the postconditioning program should be prolonged in patients prone to PIH.

Hypopigmentation is an uncommon late complication of skin resurfacing that occurs usually 6 to 12 months after the procedure. The color discrepancy may be more apparent in patients who have Fitzpatrick skin type III or greater, especially after initial erythema and PIH subside. Once the depth of resurfacing reaches the reticular dermis, permanent hypopigmentation can occur (**Fig. 7**). In most medium-depth procedures, however, true permanent hypopigmentation is rare and must be differentiated from the pseudohypopigmentation seen in photodamaged skin. Pseudohypopigmentation occurs when the newer skin is lighter than surrounding skin because of its healthier state compared with the surrounding photodamaged skin. It also can be seen temporarily in darker skinned patients until their pigment fully returns.[22]

Controlling the depth of resurfacing, carefully selecting the right candidates depending on the severity of photo damage and Fitzpatrick skin type, and resurfacing within the appropriate cosmetic units are keys to minimize the risks for apparent hypopigmentation postoperatively. When multiple facial areas need treatment, resurfacing the entire face instead of individual areas

might be a better option to avoid lines of demarcation. Alternatively, areas with the most prominent scars or rhytides can be resurfaced more deeply while areas that are not quite as damaged can be resurfaced in a lighter manner so that all the areas blend together nicely after healing is complete. Other modalities to treat postoperative hypopigmentation include the use of topical psoralen–UVA to stimulate the synthesis of melanin and the use of chemical peels to soften obvious lines of demarcation.

Scarring

One of the most devastating and serious complications of skin resurfacing is scarring. Scars can be atrophic, hypertrophic, or keloid-like and are difficult to manage (**Fig. 8**A, B). Scars often develop in areas of pruritus, prolonged erythema, delayed wound healing, or red induration. They are seen more commonly after postoperative contact dermatitis, infection, or depth of resurfacing

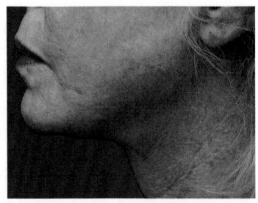

Fig. 7. Post-CO_2 laser resurfacing hypopigmentation of the cheek with a stark demarcation at the jawline where normal neck skin color is evident.

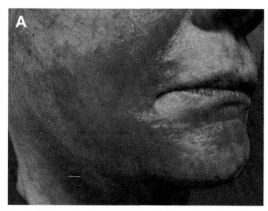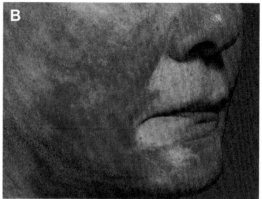

Fig. 8. (*A*) Hypertrophic and keloidal scarring after chemical peel resurfacing of the perioral area. (*B*) Same patient after a series of intralesional triamcinolone, 5-fluorouracil injections and low-fluence pulsed dye laser.

reaching the reticular dermis. Patients who have a tendency to develop keloids, a history of radiation therapy, and perioperative isotretinoin use within 6 months before the procedure or 3 months after the procedure are at increased risk for developing hypertrophic scarring.[23] In addition, certain anatomic areas, such as the neck, perioral, and periorbital regions, or areas over bony projections, such as the chin, mandibular border, and malar areas, are more prone to scar formation.[2]

Early detection and intervention are the keys to successful management of postresurfacing scars. Areas of delayed wound healing should be treated with low-level lasers or subpurpuric pulsed dye laser weekly to encourage wound healing. Areas that are healed but are indurated or very red, however, should be treated with low-level laser or pulsed dye laser in addition to the topical application of ultrapotent class I corticosteroids and silicone gel sheeting.

Microsecond 1064-nm Nd:YAG or 585-nm or 595-nm flashlamp pulsed dye laser can be used in the treatment of areas of intense erythema or hypertrophic scars to improve the color, texture, and pliability of the scar and some of its associated symptoms, such as pruritus and burning sensation. It can be performed weekly at a low to moderate setting as in the treatment of vascular lesions.[24,25] The ultrapotent topical steroid should be applied to areas of impending scars 2 days per week. If a raised or indurated scar (hypertrophic scar) already has formed, however, the topical steroid should be applied twice a day for 1 to 2 weeks and then reassessed.

Alternatively, the hypertrophic or keloidal scars can be treated with intralesional steroids if the scar does not respond to topical steroids. Close monitoring is required to monitor for the adverse effects of corticosteroids, such as telangiectasia and atrophy. The concentration of triamcinolone

acetonide used (ranging from 1 to 10 mg/mL) and the injection interval (every 2–4 weeks) are based on scar thickness. Thicker scars require more frequent injections at a higher concentration whereas thinner scars require lower concentrations. Rarely should the concentration of triamcinolone acetonide exceed 10 mg/mL. Alternatively, intralesional injections with a combination of triamcinolone acetonide and 5-fluorouracil have shown favorable results in the treatment of hypertrophic scars and keloids.[26,27]

CERTAIN COMPLICATIONS RELATED TO SPECIFIC RESURFACING MODALITIES
Complications from Deep Phenol Peels

Phenol peels cause keratolysis and keratocoagulation and can be used in various formulations, including pure phenol (88%), phenol mixed with water, or soap and croton oil (Baker-Gordon solution) to enhance the depth of penetration to skin. Because of the deeper depth of wounding caused by phenol peels, especially with Baker-Gordon solution, there is a higher incidence of prolonged erythema that can last up to 1 year followed by a high incidence of permanent hypopigmentation. Other specific complications associated with phenol peels include long-lasting (4–6 hours) intense burning sensation, cardiac arrhythmias, and laryngeal edema (**Table 1**).

Cardiac arrhythmias
Phenol is absorbed through skin, subsequently metabolized by liver, and excreted by kidneys. Patients who have impaired liver or kidney functions are more susceptible to the toxicity of phenol. In addition, the extent of cutaneous absorption of phenol is associated with the total area of exposed skin rather than the concentration of the phenol used (not related to the concentration

Table 1
The most common long-term complications specific to certain skin resurfacing modalities

Resurfacing Modality	Complications
Phenol based peels	Cardiac arrhythmias Laryngeal edema and stridor
Baker-Gordon solution	Prolonged erythema Permanent hypopigmentation Cardiac arrhythmias Laryngeal edema and stridor
Medium-depth peels	Scarring and permanent hypopigmentation (rare)
CO_2 lasers	Scarring, permanent hypopigmentation (higher incidence in older lasers)
Infrared lasers	Dermal blisters, heals with depressed scars
Microdermabrasion	Streaks of hyperpigmentation
Visible light lasers and broadband light sources	Epidermal blisters; may heal with scarring and permanent hypopigmentation
Monopolar capacitive radiofrequency	Skin blisters Permanent fat atrophy when delivered in very high energy
Plasma skin regeneration	Burns, scarring
Fractional resurfacing	Scarring Recalcitrant hyperpigmentation
Photodynamic therapy	Intra- and postoperative pain, burning sensation, edema

of phenol used). Cardiac arrhythmias, including tachycardia, premature ventricular contractions, bigeminy, paroxysmal atrial tachycardia, ventricular tachycardia, and atrial fibrillation, can be seen in phenol-based peels with rapid application in the full-face treatment.[28–30] It is important, therefore, to use cardiac monitoring during the resurfacing procedure and in the recovery period, allowing for immediate detection of potential cardiac complications. Pausing for 15 minutes between applications of phenol-based peels to each cosmetic unit that allows a total of 60 to 90 minutes for the whole procedure is recommended to allow ongoing metabolism when treating the entire face.[12,31] Many surgeons also preload patients with intravenous fluids to facilitate the metabolism of phenol and renal clearance, thus avoiding a toxic systemic dose.

Laryngeal edema

Laryngeal edema is an uncommon complication in patients undergoing phenol peels. Klein and Little[32] reported that 3 of 245 female patients developed laryngeal edema along with stridor, hoarseness, and tachypnea within 24 hours after phenol peeling that resolved within another 24 hours after heated mist inhalation therapy. All three patients were heavy smokers. Probable mechanisms of this complication include possible additive effects of irritation to larynx by ether fumes and cigarette smoke or a hypersensitivity reaction to phenol.

Complications from Microdermabrasion

Microdermabrasion has become extremely popular and is estimated to be the second most performed cosmetic procedure by the American Academy of Cosmetic Surgery.[33] Compared with dermabrasion and chemical peels, this procedure intends to create gentle superficial mechanical abrasion of the skin to the depth of the upper epidermis only. It generally is considered as a safe procedure with minimal adverse effects. Complications can happen with microdermabrasion, however. Abrasions from improperly performed procedures can result in pinpoint bleeding, petechia, purpura, and streaks of PIH once they heal, if the depth of wounding reaches the papillary dermis or the negative pressure of the handpiece is too intense.[34]

An unusual case of an acute urticarial response occurring immediately after microdermabrasion was reported by Farris and Rietschel.[35] In this report, a patient had known allergy to latex and a history of dermatographism. The particles of microdermabrasion were aluminum oxide crystals. This patient developed pruritus and urticarial plaques within 2 minutes after the procedure to the neck and face. She was given diphenhydramine and intramuscular betamethasone dipropionate and later received systemic corticosteroids after developing "fullness in the throat." Possible causes of this severe acute urticarial response included exposure to latex from microdermabrasion unit, exaggerated dermographism, or pressure-induced urticaria.

Other complications associated with microdermabrasion, including ocular irritation, chemosis, photophobia, and punctate keratitis, can occur if aluminum oxide crystals enter the eyes; therefore, protective ocular shields are recommended during the procedure.[36]

Complications from Ablative and Nonablative Laser Resurfacing

Ablative laser skin resurfacing

The CO_2 laser and the erbium (Er):YAG laser are the two main modalities used in ablative laser skin resurfacing. The penetration depth of the Er:YAG laser is approximately 1 to 3 μm of tissue per J/cm^2 whereas that of CO_2 laser reaches 20 to 30 μm. Thus, the Er:YAG laser has a more precise ablation and causes minimal thermal damage to surrounding tissues compared with the CO_2 laser and provides less tissue contraction or tightening than the CO_2 laser.[15,37] The residual thermal damage that extends and deeper depth of dermal coagulation, however, result in more tissue tightening, making the CO_2 laser an overall superior modality in ablative resurfacing.[38] Because the depth of wounding reaches the reticular dermis, the rates of permanent hypopigmentation and scarring are increased significantly with the CO_2 laser resurfacing. The incidence and severity of other adverse effects, such as immediate edema, oozing, tissue crusting, and prolonged erythema, also are higher in the CO_2 laser resurfacing. These adverse effects are seen more commonly, especially in the continuous wave CO_2 laser that was used in the 1980s and 1990s. Therefore, newer generation of CO_2 lasers, including high-pulsed or scanned CO_2 lasers, were developed with the capability of delivering high peak powers with short pulses and rapid movement across the skin surface. This provides more precise control of the depth of ablation and selective thermal damage, significantly reducing the rate of severe side effects, such as prolonged erythema, permanent hypopigmentation, and scarring, without compromising efficacy.[39–41] Furthermore, the development of blended lasers (CO_2 and Er:YAG) and tunable pulse duration Er:YAG lasers have made these laser modalities safer.

Nonablative laser resurfacing

Nonablative laser resurfacing can stimulate collagen production and tissue remodeling and improve texture and dyschromia in a noninvasive approach that causes less discomfort to patients and has minimal downtime.

Commonly used infrared (IR) laser systems for nonablative laser skin resurfacing include 1320-nm Nd:YAG laser, 1450-nm diode laser, 1540-nm Er:glass laser, and 2790-nm Er:yttrium-scandium-gallium-garnet (YSGG) laser. They target the dermis by causing selective dermal injury to improve the skin texture whereas epidermis protection is achieved by concomitant cooling. In general, the higher the frequency used, the greater the degree of clinical improvement is achieved. Because most energy is delivered to the dermis with epidermal protection, dermal blisters caused by dermal swelling without epidermal changes can be seen in IR laser resurfacing. These dermal blisters can heal with depressed scars. Epidermal blisters also can be associated with IR laser resurfacing but are less common (**Fig. 9**).

Visible lasers and broadband light sources, such as the pulsed dye laser (585 nm or 595 nm), pulsed 532-nm potassium titanyl phosphate laser, and intense pulsed light sources, are widely used in the treatment of red and brown discolorations. The chromophores are hemoglobin or melanin. Epidermal blisters can occur as a result of melanin absorption when high energy is delivered (**Fig. 10**).

Monopolar and bipolar radiofrequency is a promising technology that tightens skin and soft tissue in a nonablative approach. It delivers a uniform volumetric energy into the reticular dermis and underlying tissue. The heat is generated by the resistance of the tissue to the current flow, subsequently inducing partial collagen denaturation, collagen shrinkage, and skin tightening with minimal epidermal injury.[42] The most common complications include minimal transient erythema and mild edema that usually resolve

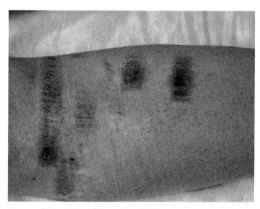

Fig. 9. Blistering after semiablative laser resurfacing with a fractionated 1540-nm Er:glass laser.

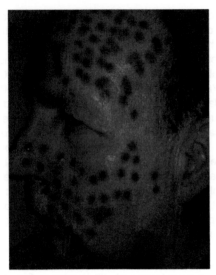

Fig. 10. Diffuse blistering incurred by pulsed dye laser on tanned skin. This resulted in permanent hypopigmentation in certain areas.

spontaneously within 1 to 2 days after the radiofrequency treatment. Other complications, such as persistent edema, superficial skin burns, and skin blisters, are more likely to occur at higher energy settings.[43] Patients also may experience temporary numbness of the skin, which is innervated by the greater auricular nerve. No permanent damage of the nerve has been reported.[44] One of the most serious complications is permanent fat atrophy that can occur when high energy is delivered during treatments.[45] Therefore, multiple passes at lower-energy settings is the key treatment algorithm to accomplish an optimal tightening result and to avoid permanent fat atrophy.

Plasma Skin Regeneration (Semiablative)

Plasma skin regeneration is a novel technology that generates pulses of ultrahigh frequency energy that convert nitrogen gas into plasma within the handpiece which is subsequently delivered to the area of treatment. The rapid heating generated through the excited gas then is transferred to the skin resulting in epidermal necrosis and increased dermal collagen production. Skin burns with erythema, edema, and desquamation of epidermis are common side effects of this procedure. Depending on the depth of the wounding, scarring can be a potential risk associated with plasma skin regeneration.[46]

Fractional Resurfacing (Semiablative)

Fractional photothermolysis creates noncontiguous columns of microthermal zones in the dermis.

Each microcolumn generates a localized zone of epidermal necrosis and collagen denaturation because of the thermal injury, whereas tissues surrounding each column are spared, resulting in rapid epidermal regeneration.

In general, fractional resurfacing has a significantly lower rate of complications compared with traditional ablative resurfacing. As the depth of the penetration is energy dependent, however, there is a potential risk for hypertrophic scarring if bulk heating is delivered to the area of treatment. Common complications include a transient burning sensation, mild sunburn-like erythema, and postoperative edema that usually is mild and resolves spontaneously within several days after the procedure. Other common complications that can be seen in any resurfacing procedure include acneiform eruptions, purpura, postinflammatory hyperpigmentation, prolonged erythema, reactivation of HSV, dermatitis, and bacterial infections.[47] Sixty percent of patients may experience flaking and approximately 87% of patients may have xerosis. Bronzing also can occur 3 days postoperatively that often lasts for 3 to 4 days.[48] Based on the author's (Obagi's) experience, an unusual type of recalcitrant hyperpigmentation (**Fig. 11**) that is resistant to topical bleaching agents, superficial chemical peels, and microdermabrasion also is seen with fractional photothermolysis (personal communication, Suzan Obagi, 2008). Patients who have this condition tend to have darker skin phenotypes and melasma.

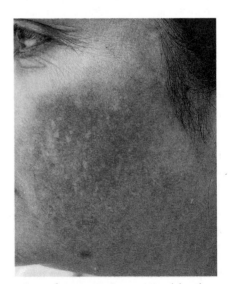

Fig. 11. One of many patients treated by the senior physician for acne scars and melasma with subsequent persistent and recalcitrant hyperpigmentation after fractional laser ablation using a 1540-nm Er:glass laser.

Photodynamic therapy

PDT involves topical application of a photosensitizer, which accumulates selectively in cells with elevated metabolism. When the light is shined at a wavelength that activates the photosensitizer, singlet oxygen and free radicals are produced leading to cellular destruction and photorejuvenation by affecting extra cellular matrix components. Common side effects associated with PDT are uncommon but include pain and burning sensation during the procedure, postoperative erythema, scaling, crusting, postoperative pain, and edema (related to length of application of 5-aminolevulinic acid or other photosensitizers).[49] Allergic contact dermatitis to methyl aminolevulinate also is reported after PDT treatment.[50]

SUMMARY

In conclusion, the field of skin resurfacing is undergoing rapid evolution with many new technologies that have developed, providing more choices for physicians and patients. Knowing the potential adverse effects associated with each skin resurfacing modality is paramount in selecting the appropriate approach for each candidate, thereby minimizing complications and achieving optimal results.

REFERENCES

1. Alster TS. Cutaneous resurfacing with CO_2 and erbium: YAG lasers: preoperative, intraoperative, and postoperative considerations. Plast Reconstr Surg 1999;103:619–32 [discussion 633–14].
2. Nanni CA, Alster TS. Complications of carbon dioxide laser resurfacing. An evaluation of 500 patients. Dermatol Surg 1998;24:315–20.
3. Bernstein LJ, Kauvar AN, Grossman MC, et al. The short- and long-term side effects of carbon dioxide laser resurfacing. Dermatol Surg 1997;23:519–25.
4. Sriprachya-Anunt S, Fitzpatrick RE, Goldman MP, et al. Infections complicating pulsed carbon dioxide laser resurfacing for photoaged facial skin. Dermatol Surg 1997;23:527–35 [discussion 535–26].
5. Walia S, Alster TS. Cutaneous CO_2 laser resurfacing infection rate with and without prophylactic antibiotics. Dermatol Surg 1999;25:857–61.
6. Demas PN, Bridenstine JB. Diagnosis and treatment of postoperative complications after skin resurfacing. J Oral Maxillofac Surg 1999;57:837–41.
7. Asken S. Unoccluded Baker-Gordon phenol peels—review and update. J Dermatol Surg Oncol 1989;15:998–1008.
8. Beeson WH, Rachel JD. Valacyclovir prophylaxis for herpes simplex virus infection or infection

9. Alster TS, Nanni CA. Famciclovir prophylaxis of herpes simplex virus reactivation after laser skin resurfacing. Dermatol Surg 1999;25:242–6.
10. Rao J, Golden TA, Fitzpatrick RE. Atypical mycobacterial infection following blepharoplasty and full-face skin resurfacing with CO2 laser. Dermatol Surg 2002;28:768–71 [discussion 771].
11. Weinstein C. Carbon dioxide laser resurfacing. Long-term follow-up in 2123 patients. Clin Plast Surg 1998;25:109–30.
12. Brody HJ. Complications of chemical resurfacing. Dermatol Clin 2001;19:427–38, vii–viii.
13. Weinstein C, Ramirez OM, Pozner JN. Postoperative care following CO_2 laser resurfacing: avoiding pitfalls. Plast Reconstr Surg 1997;100:1855–66.
14. Langsdon PR, Milburn M, Yarber R. Comparison of the laser and phenol chemical peel in facial skin resurfacing. Arch Otolaryngol Head Neck Surg 2000;126:1195–9.
15. Alexiades-Armenakas MR, Dover JS, Arndt KA. The spectrum of laser skin resurfacing: nonablative, fractional, and ablative laser resurfacing. J Am Acad Dermatol 2008;58:719–37 [quiz 738–740].
16. Rapaport MJ, Rapaport V. Prolonged erythema after facial laser resurfacing or phenol peel secondary to corticosteroid addiction. Dermatol Surg 1999;25:781–4 [discussion 785].
17. Lowe NJ, Lask G, Griffin ME. Laser skin resurfacing. Pre- and posttreatment guidelines. Dermatol Surg 1995;21:1017–9.
18. Obagi ZE. Skin classification. In: Obagi ZE, editor. Obagi skin health restoration and rejuvenation. New York: Springer-Verlag; 2000. p. 65–85.
19. Ho C, Nguyen Q, Lowe NJ, et al. Laser resurfacing in pigmented skin. Dermatol Surg 1995;21:1035–7.
20. Horton S, Alster TS. Preoperative and postoperative considerations for carbon dioxide laser resurfacing. Cutis 1999;64:399–406.
21. Obagi S. Pre- and postlaser skin care. Oral Maxillofac Surg Clin North Am 2004;16(2):181–7.
22. Alster TS, Lupton JR. Prevention and treatment of side effects and complications of cutaneous laser resurfacing. Plast Reconstr Surg 2002;109:308–16 [discussion 317–08].
23. Katz BE, Mac Farlane DF. Atypical facial scarring after isotretinoin therapy in a patient with previous dermabrasion. J Am Acad Dermatol 1994;30:852–3.
24. Dierickx C, Goldman MP, Fitzpatrick RE. Laser treatment of erythematous/hypertrophic and pigmented scars in 26 patients. Plast Reconstr Surg 1995;95:84–90 [discussion 91–82].
25. Alster TS, Williams CM. Treatment of keloid sternotomy scars with 585 nm flashlamp-pumped pulsed-dye laser. Lancet 1995;345:1198–200.

26. Asilian A, Darougheh A, Shariati F. New combination of triamcinolone, 5-Fluorouracil, and pulsed-dye laser for treatment of keloid and hypertrophic scars. Dermatol Surg 2006;32:907–15.

27. Goldan O, Weissman O, Regev E, et al. Treatment of postdermabrasion facial hypertrophic and keloid scars with intralesional 5-Fluorouracil injections. Aesthetic Plast Surg 2008;32:389–92.

28. Landau M. Cardiac complications in deep chemical peels. Dermatol Surg 2007;33:190–3 [discussion 193].

29. Gross BG. Cardiac arrhythmias during phenol face peeling. Plast Reconstr Surg 1984;73:590–4.

30. Truppman ES, Ellenby JD. Major electrocardiographic changes during chemical face peeling. Plast Reconstr Surg 1979;63:44–8.

31. Beeson WH. The importance of cardiac monitoring in superficial and deep chemical peeling. J Dermatol Surg Oncol 1987;13:949–50.

32. Klein DR, Little JH. Laryngeal edema as a complication of chemical peel. Plast Reconstr Surg 1983;71:419–20.

33. Hernandez-Perez E, Ibiett EV. Gross and microscopic findings in patients undergoing microdermabrasion for facial rejuvenation. Dermatol Surg 2001;27:637–40.

34. Grimes PE. Microdermabrasion. Dermatol Surg 2005;31:1160–5 [discussion 1165].

35. Farris PK, Rietschel RL. An unusual acute urticarial response following microdermabrasion. Dermatol Surg 2002;28:606–8 [discussion 608].

36. Morgenstern KE, Foster JA. Advances in cosmetic oculoplastic surgery. Curr Opin Ophthalmol 2002;13:324–30.

37. Ross EV, McKinlay JR, Anderson RR. Why does carbon dioxide resurfacing work? A review. Arch Dermatol 1999;135:444–54.

38. Walsh JT Jr, Deutsch TF. Pulsed CO_2 laser tissue ablation: measurement of the ablation rate. Lasers Surg Med 1988;8:264–75.

39. Alster TS, Garg S. Treatment of facial rhytides with a high-energy pulsed carbon dioxide laser. Plast Reconstr Surg 1996;98:791–4.

40. Alster TS. Comparison of two high-energy, pulsed carbon dioxide lasers in the treatment of periorbital rhytides. Dermatol Surg 1996;22:541–5.

41. Apfelberg DB. A critical appraisal of high-energy pulsed carbon dioxide laser facial resurfacing for acne scars. Ann Plast Surg 1997;38:95–100.

42. Zelickson BD, Kist D, Bernstein E, et al. Histological and ultrastructural evaluation of the effects of a radiofrequency-based nonablative dermal remodeling device: a pilot study. Arch Dermatol 2004;140:204–9.

43. Fitzpatrick R, Geronemus R, Goldberg D, et al. Multicenter study of noninvasive radiofrequency for periorbital tissue tightening. Lasers Surg Med 2003;33:232–42.

44. Abraham MT, Vic Ross E. Current concepts in nonablative radiofrequency rejuvenation of the lower face and neck. Facial Plast Surg 2005;21:65–73.

45. Abraham MT, Chiang SK, Keller GS, et al. Clinical evaluation of non-ablative radiofrequency facial rejuvenation. J Cosmet Laser Ther 2004;6:136–44.

46. Alster TS, Konda S. Plasma skin resurfacing for regeneration of neck, chest, and hands: investigation of a novel device. Dermatol Surg 2007;33:1315–21.

47. Graber EM, Tanzi EL, Alster TS. Side effects and complications of fractional laser photothermolysis: experience with 961 treatments. Dermatol Surg 2008;34:301–5 [discussion 305–7].

48. Tannous Z. Fractional resurfacing. Clin Dermatol 2007;25:480–6.

49. Redbord KP, Hanke CW. Topical photodynamic therapy for dermatologic disorders: results and complications. J Drugs Dermatol 2007;6:1197–202.

50. Hohwy T, Andersen KE, Solvsten H, et al. Allergic contact dermatitis to methyl aminolevulinate after photodynamic therapy in 9 patients. Contact Derm 2007;57:321–3.

Complications in Fillers and Botox

Joseph Niamtu III, DMD

KEYWORDS

- Botox • Injectable fillers • Botox complications
- Filler complications • Injectable filler complications
- Minimally invasive cosmetic facial surgery
- Facial wrinkle improvement

Americans spent $11 billion on cosmetic surgery procedures in 2007. Almost 3 billion of those dollars were spent on minimally invasive procedures, of which injectable facial fillers and botulinum toxin type A (Botox) were the most popular. Injectables (fillers and Botox) have fueled the fires of the popularity of cosmetic facial surgery. They have provided more options to patients and surgeons and provided quick, affordable, predictable, and long-lasting improvement of facial wrinkles and lip augmentation. Even in sour economies, patients want to look good and although they may not have money to spend on surgical procedures, injectable treatments remain popular. This article addresses common complications of injectable fillers and Botox.

COMPLICATIONS OF BOTOX TREATMENT

At the time of this writing, Botox and botulinum toxin type B (Myobloc) are the only neurotoxins approved by the Food and Drug Administration. Also, at the time of this writing, there are nine other neurotoxins in review for Food and Drug Administration approval. The more correct word for this group of drugs is neuromodulators, which better describes their action.

The mechanism of Botox is to prevent the release of acetylcholine at the motor end plate. Without this release, the electrical impulse is not transmitted; hence, the muscle does not move. Selective paralysis is the keystone of neuromodulator treatment but only if the toxin is in the anticipated and desired location.

When discussing complications of Botox cosmetic procedures, complications must be differentiated from sequellae. A true complication is upper eyelid ptosis, for example, whereas failure to respond to an injection sequence is a sequella. **Box 1** lists some common complications or sequellae of Botox treatment.

Undertreatment

There is threshold at which Botox is effective. I believe that some patients simply are more sensitive than others to the drug's effect. For 12 years I have used 20 units of Botox per treatment area (glabella, frontalis, or lateral canthus) with an estimated 95% success rate for patient satisfaction. Every injector experiences patients who return to the office after Botox injection and report that "my Botox did not work." Some of these patients are adamant and disgruntled and request free retreatment or refund. This can be an unpleasant situation but easily is prevented by adequate preinjection discussion and proper informed consent. It is important for patients to realize that some patients are sensitive to Botox and some are resistant or immune. I have been told that a past subclinical botulinum infection from food poisoning that did not require hospitalization could cause an immunity to botulinum toxin type A. Secondary to that, some patients simply do not respond to any amount of the toxin. I once had a nurse who was resistant to 40 units of Botox in the glabella. The Botox representative provided free Botox and another 20 units was given, still with no result, not even a little. I subsequently treated the patient

Cosmetic Facial Surgery, 11319 Polo Place, Midlothian, VA 23113, USA
E-mail address: niamtu@niamtu.com

Oral Maxillofacial Surg Clin N Am 21 (2009) 13–21
doi:10.1016/j.coms.2008.11.001
1042-3699/08/$ – see front matter © 2009 Elsevier Inc. All rights reserved.

oralmaxsurgery.theclinics.com

**Box 1
Common complications of Botox treatment**

Overcorrection

Undercorrection

Asymmetric result

Upper eyelid ptosis

Dysphagia, neck weakness

Perioral droop

Compromised result in elderly

Bruising

Intravascular injection

Lagophthalmous, exposure keratosis

Globe perforation

Diplopia (lateral rectus)

Psychosomatic problems

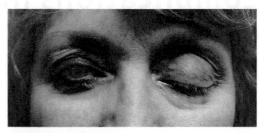

Fig. 2. This patient was injected at another office and experienced severe upper eyelid ptosis lasting 10 weeks.

with botulinum toxin type B, which still did little to stop her muscle movement. This is a rare occurrence among the thousands of patients I have treated for 12 years.

Overtreatment

When Botox first came on the scene, the trend was for doctors and patients to aim for a treatment goal of total paralysis. In the early days, patients complained at the least bit of forehead or glabellar movement. This "frozen face" appearance came to be disdained by patients and contemporary treatment goals are relaxing or softening the muscle movement. Overtreating any area can produce unnatural animation, which patients do not like. My personal words of wisdom to novice injectors are,

"always be conservative as you can always add more Botox, but you can't take it away or turn it off." Having said this, I believe patients should understand that Botox treatment is a sculpting process and that returning to the office 1 to 2 weeks after the first series on injections is a good thing so that they can be precision treated or adjusted.

The biggest problem I have witnessed in my practice and that of colleagues is overtreatment of the frontalis in female patients who have upper lid skin excess. The problem is as follows. Many women unconsciously lift their eyebrows (any surgeon who performs brow lift surgery and tries to get prospective patients to relax their brows can testify to this), which elevates the excess skin of the upper eyelid. If the frontalis is heavily treated (especially the lateral areas) the main brow elevator is deactivated. When this happens, patients who usually lift their lids no longer can, making the brow and lid feel heavy and, because the brow is not elevated, the excess upper lid skin is more apparent. Classically this occurs on approximately the third postinjection day, when patients apply eye shadow to their upper lids and cannot elevate them. Next, patients go to the Internet to

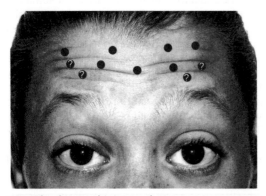

Fig. 1. The dots on this image show a common pattern for frontalis injection. The question marks indicate areas to avoid or to inject conservatively in patients who have upper lid excess.

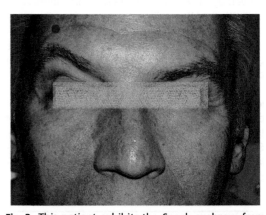

Fig. 3. This patient exhibits the Spock eyebrow from undertreatment of the lateral frontalis. The black circle illustrates the area to retreat to correct the problem.

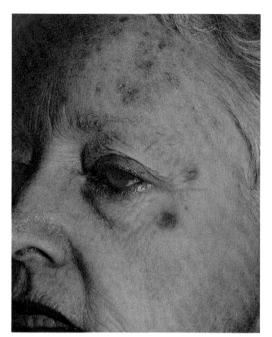

Fig. 4. When a patient comes to a doctor to look better and leaves with a bruise, the impact is negative.

> **Box 2**
> **Common filler complications**
>
> Unrealistic patient expectations
> Bruising/hematoma
> Undercorrection
> Overcorrection
> Asymmetry
> Lumping
> Iatrogenic factors
> Allergic reaction

True Eyelid Ptosis

Thankfully true ptosis is a rare and usually novice complication. Eyelid opening is controlled by the levator palpebrae superiorus muscle, which in turn inserts into the levator aponeurosis of the upper eyelid. If Botox is injected (or more commonly diffuses) into this muscle, the eyelid does not open (**Fig. 2**). Albeit temporary, this is a huge problem for patients as it not only affects their appearance in a negative way but also may make simple tasks, such as reading and driving, impossible. This complication can be avoided by keeping all injections at least 1 cm above the bony orbital rim. Some teachers recommend injecting just beneath the brow. This is acceptable if patients have normal positioned brows, but in patients who have ptotic brows, the injection may be close to the levator muscle. Injecting 1 cm above the orbital rim is a pearl that has kept this author from producing upper lid ptosis over the past 12 years. Drops of Iopidine 0.5%

search out Botox complications and then accuse the injector of "drooping their eyelid." In reality, their eyelid function is fine; the problem is that they cannot elevate their brow as they have been used to and, because of that, the upper eyelid skin appears excessive. The antidote to this situation is to treat the lateral frontalis conservatively in older patients who have dermatochalasis and protect with informed consent and preinjection consultation **Fig. 1**.

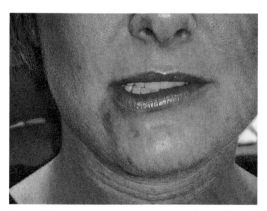

Fig. 5. This patient was treated at another office for the DAO but the lip depressors (likely the depressor labii) were affected. The patient's left side is affected in this image.

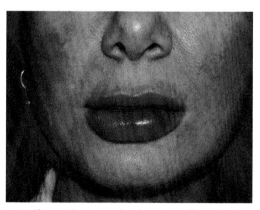

Fig. 6. This patient was developed swelling, bruising, and minor hematoma immediately after filler injection.

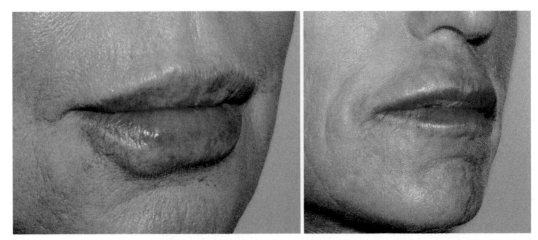

Fig. 7. These patients treated at other offices show not only overfill but also incorrect placement of the filler in the lips.

stimulate Müller's muscle and provide several millimeters of lid opening to assist the problem. The effects of the drops are not long lasting and usually are applied before social interaction to slightly open the affected lid. Although not a "cure," it can assist a distraught patient.

Another periorbital muscle problem involves Botox diffusion into the extraocular muscles, namely the lateral rectus muscle. Diplopia can result and has resulted from paralysis of the lateral

rectus muscle. Again, staying 1 cm lateral to the orbital rim prevents this problem in my experience.

Some practitioners recommend not lying down, working out, or performing other strenuous activity for 4 hours after Botox injection to prevent septal diffusion leading to ptosis. Although I used to recommend this, I stopped approximately 5 years ago and now tell patients to do anything they want post injection. I have yet to see a complication from that.

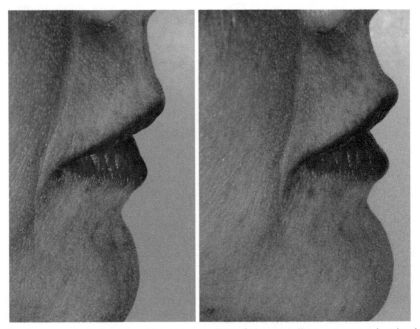

Fig. 8. This patient was treated properly with augmentation of the vermillion-cutaneous border, but the deep vermillion was undertreated and should have been augmented with enough filler to increase the pout and projection of the lips.

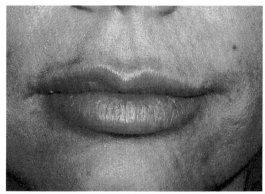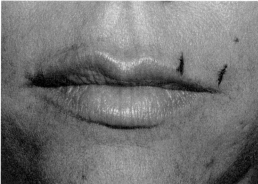

Fig. 9. This patient exhibited asymmetry from undertreatment of her left side. The marked area indicates where the touch up filler was needed.

Asymmetry

Asymmetric treatment results are not uncommon and can be a result of injector placement or patient anatomic variation. One of the most common asymmetries is the Spock eyebrow. This is a demonic curvature of the lateral brow that occurs when the central frontalis is deactivated but the lateral frontalis is active and only lifts the brow tail (**Fig. 3**). This is easily corrected by placing some additional Botox at the active area on the frontalis.

Bruising

Postinjection ecchymosis is a phenomenon that even the most experienced injectors occasionally see (**Fig. 4**). This occurs when a vessel is disrupted by the injection needle. Using a 32-gauge needle and paying close attention to the superficial vasculature can limit this situation. The most common area for bruising is the lateral canthus region where the skin is thin and the veins superficial.

Besides the outward negative cosmetic effect of a bruise, women who have facial bruises may lead others to assume spousal abuse may have occurred. Finally, many women do not tell their significant others that they are spending money on Botox and the bruise is difficult to explain. Screening patients for aspirin or other drugs that affect platelet aggregation also is important in preventing bruising.

Perioral Droop

Injecting Botox in the lips to address vertical rhytids, injecting the depressor anguli oris (DAO) to upturn the corners of the mouth, and injecting the mentalis to address skin puckering of the chin have become commonly requested treatments. Injecting the lower face is more tenuous

in terms of complications that the upper face. Lip, DAO, and mentalis injections all can cause or contribute to dysfunctional animation of the perioral region (**Fig. 5**). The best treatment for this is prevention. Again, a patient who presents to a cosmetic office to look better but is left drooling, lisping, or with the inability to pucker will not be happy. Lower facial Botox treatment should be reserved for advanced injectors and conservative treatment should be a mantra. Remember, more Botox always can be added but cannot be taken away.

Unrealistic Patient Expectations

Although not a complication, an unhappy patient is a problem. If patients are injected and return with an incomplete treatment (residual muscle movement), they may want free retreatment or refund. This is common especially when an office charges by the area. Patients pay a certain amount for glabellar treatment and when they return with residual muscle movement, they expect the doctor to be

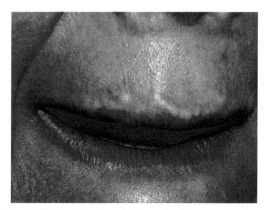

Fig. 10. This patient was injected with a particulate filler that not only was improperly placed as interrupted boluses but also was not blended by massaging.

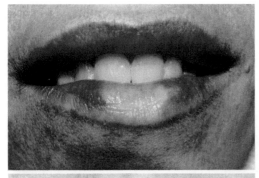

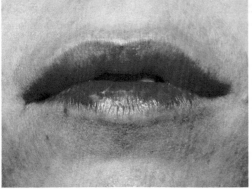

Fig. 11. Blanching should alert the injector that the filler may be placed too superficially. Blanching is usually self-limiting as shown in the bottom picture, but if too much pressure is placed on the tissue, necrosis can result.

COMPLICATIONS OF INJECTABLE FACIAL FILLERS

Like Botox, injectable fillers are one of the most requested minimally invasive cosmetic procedures. In theory they are simple—plumping up wrinkles or lips by injecting a volume of fillers. As simple as they seem, however, the learning curve of fillers is steep. Anyone can inject, but only experienced injectors can make magic. The number one rule for fillers is the same as for Botox and for all cosmetic procedures: be conservative, start with appetizer portions, and encourage patients to return for postinjection follow-up. I explain to my patients that filler treatment is a sculpting process and sometimes requires more than one injection session to get the job done right. It can be considered a quality control process. Many times I have been happy with the immediate injection result but when patients return at 2 weeks, I am not happy. Sometimes patients are happy at follow-up, but I know the results can be better. A subtle asymmetry or other problem that would pass as acceptable to an untrained eye can affect my reputation among professionals. Unfavorable cosmetic surgery cannot be hidden, so it pays to follow-up treatments.

When considering the possible complications of filler treatment, an entire text could be written; however, the most common problems are discussed in this article (**Box 2**).

Unrealistic Patient Expectations

As with any cosmetic procedure, a problem can be patients expecting too much or surgeons failing to discuss a procedure and details adequately. Older patients who have atrophic lips, smoker's lines, and perioral wrinkles cannot be led to believe

responsible for it. As discussed previously, preinjection discussion and informed consent should cover this. When practitioners charge by the unit instead of the area, it is a cut-and-dried decision as to patients needing more Botox—they simply pay for the extra units.

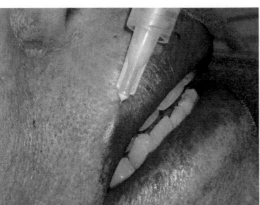

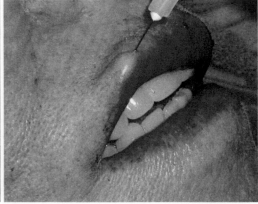

Fig. 12. The correct needle placement for white roll (vermilion-cutaneous) outlining is in the potential space between the mucosa and muscle at the skin vermillion interface. The top image shows the proper placement whereas the bottom image shows the filler clumping in a ball from a too superficial injection.

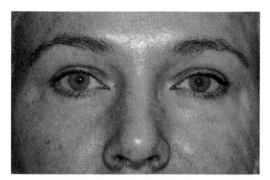

Fig. 13. The bluish tinge of a clear hyaluronic acid filler is seen in the lower lids of this patient injected for tear trough deformity.

they will leave with voluptuous lips. They can be improved, but underpromising is a good idea.

Some patients also have unrealistic expectations about such things as how long fillers last and degree of correction. Experienced injectors use common sense, before and after pictures, and informed consent to present a realistic expectation for patients.

Bruising/Hematoma

Bruising/hematoma is a harmless but disconcerting problem for patients and surgeons. Patients present to look better and leave looking worse. The lips and perioral areas are vascular and even the best injectors on occasion experience bruising and, less frequently, hematoma. Making sure that patients are not taking any substances that effect platelet aggregation is a primary consideration.

Also, icing the lips before and immediately after injection is helpful. **Fig. 6** shows bruising or hematoma that can occur with facial fillers. These areas are treated initially with ice, then with heat.

Undertreatment

Undertreatment is a relative complication and the best one to have if there is choice. Undertreatment occurs when inadequate filler is placed and the result is less than desired. This can be a true undertreatment or a patient-centered situation. Underfilling lips or wrinkles, other than the inconvenience to patients, generally is a problem as they simply require more filler. A patient-centered situation refers to situations that occur when patients decline to purchase the correct amount of filler required to fill a defect adequately. Over the years I have declined to treat nasolabial folds in adults who have had a single syringe of filler. Many patients want to economize and only want to purchase a single syringe of filler. For anyone over age 40, this generally is inadequate volume to do the job. By trying to "split" a syringe on each side, there is not enough filler to complete the correction. What remains is a substandard treatment and a disappointed patient. When patients request this, I politely ask them to save their money and return when we can do the procedure correctly. This has paid off in excellent treatment results. The situation is that deeper folds need more filler and there is no better experience than a patient who can afford to use as much filler as necessary to achieve the maximum aesthetic result.

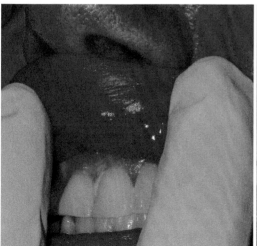
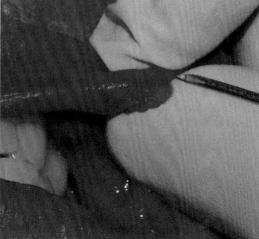

Fig. 14. This patient was treated improperly at another office. The lump of superficial filler is nicked with an 18-gauge needle and expressed by compressing the surrounding tissue.

Overtreatment

Overtreatment is a problem that definitely makes unhappy patients. Patients seek filler injection for a natural correction and an overaugmented result calls attention to the result, which is aggravating to patients and surgeons. The best way to avoid overcorrection is to be conservative. As discussed previously, there is nothing wrong with a second session. Depending on the filler, it is possible to reverse the result. Hyaluronidase dissolves the hyaluronic acid fillers. Although permanent fillers sound like a great idea to patients, when overfilled, sometimes surgery is required to correct the problem. Great care must be taken when using longer-lasting or permanent fillers. **Figs. 7** and **8** show two patients not only who were overtreated but also whose filler was placed in the incorrect tissue plane or area of the lip.

Asymmetry

Asymmetry is a situation of overcorrection of one side or undercorrection of the other. This sometimes is not noticed at the actual treatment because of tissue edema, especially with the hydrophilic hyaluronic acid fillers. This is why it is important to follow-up filler patients. The patient pictured in **Fig. 9** was adequately treated for vermillion border fill but undertreated on her left side.

Lumping

One of the most common novice problems is an inhomogeneous placement of the filler material. Massage is just as important as filler placement in my opinion. The filler is placed in small spheres or strands and is fluid in the tissues. By massaging the injected areas, the filler is compacted and blended to form a more contiguous and smooth texture. Failure to do this can lead to palpable and visible irregularities (**Fig. 10**).

Iatrogenic Factors

Technically, all the complications discussed previously may be classified as iatrogenic (the fault of the operator). Injecting in the incorrect tissue plane is a good example of a physician-induced problem. Most fillers are intradermal, and, although this exact tissue plane is debatable, fillers frequently are injected too deeply or too superficially. When teaching new injectors, I tell them that they should be able to see a wrinkle or fold improve as they are injecting or they are in the wrong plane. It also is important to realize the proper plane of injection for each specific filler as the particles are designed to be placed in specific planes. Some are superficial dermal, most are

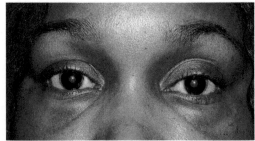
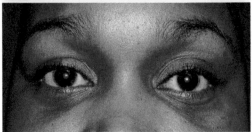

Fig. 15. This patient was injected with hyaluronic acid filler for tear trough correction and the filler was injected too superficially (*top image*). The same patient is shown 24 hours later (*lower image*) after injecting 70 units of hyaluronidase (diluted with local anesthetic) in each lower lid in the area of the filler excess.

mid-dermal, and others are subcutaneous. Injecting too deep simply wastes filler and does not properly plump the wrinkle. Injecting too superficially makes the contour irregular or even necroses the tissue. **Fig. 11** shows blanching from a filler injection that is too superficial. When an injector sees blanching, the needle should be redirected as the blanching could cause necrosis from disruption of the surrounding vasculature.

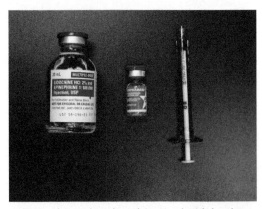

Fig. 16. Hyaluronidase (1 mL) is mixed with local anesthetic (1 mL) for a total of 150 units per 2 mL; 1 mL (70 units) is injected in areas of significant filler whereas smaller amounts are used for less significant filler excess.

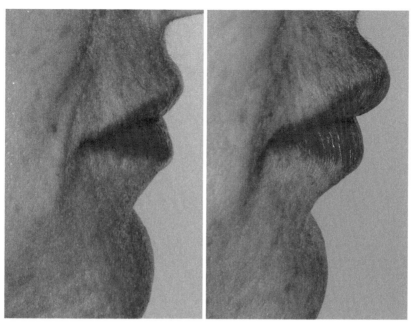

Fig. 17. This patient is shown before and immediately after injection of hyaluronic acid filler (0.4 mL) in each lip. Significant and immediate swelling occurred but resolved spontaneously within 48 hours.

When injecting the lips, two planes are involved. For white roll or Cupid's bow definition, the filler is injected into the potential space between the mucosa and muscle. When a needle is in this correct plane, the syringe pressure should be easy and the filler should flow antegrade and retrograde making a well-formed outline. If a needle is too superficial, the syringe pressure is increased and the filler clumps up in a ball instead of flowing freely along the vermilion-cutaneous border (**Fig. 12**).

Given the popularity of hyaluronic acid fillers, the Tyndall effect (or similar phenomenon) commonly is seen, especially in areas of thin skin. The Tyndall effect is a situation where a clear filler appears blue under the skin. This can be seen in any dermal region but is particularly common in the thin lower eyelid skin in white patients (**Fig. 13**). In the tear trough region, the filler should be placed at the periosteal lever or at least in the suborbicularis oculi plane.

Getting rid of or reducing unwanted filler can be achieved by several means. For excess superficial filler, sometimes making a stab incision with an 18-gauge needle and expressing the excess filler are all that is necessary (**Fig. 14**).

One insurance policy when using hyaluronic acid fillers is the ability to reduce or reverse them with hyaluronidase. Hyaluronidase hydrolyzes the hyaluronic acid in a matter of hours. The hyaluronidase is mixed with saline or local anesthetic and then injected into the region of excess filler. I generally use approximately 70 units of hyaluronidase to reverse significant excess and a smaller amount for less severe overcorrections. A small amount, approximately 20 units, may be used to slightly reduce excess whereas large amounts totally reverse the result. Sometimes patients want all the filler dissolved and other times just want the specific area reduced. There is little danger in placing too much hyaluronidase in an area. The substance also dissolves some of the native tissue hyaluronidase, but this is replenished within 24 hours. **Fig. 15** shows a patient who was overtreated in the tear trough region (top image) and the same patient 24 hours later after injecting 70 units of hyaluronidase in each lower lid in the plane the filler was placed. **Fig. 16** shows the materials used to dissolve hyaluronic acid fillers.

Allergic Reaction

True allergic reaction is rare and most fillers no longer require allergy testing. Any patient can be allergic to some component of any filler. Some reactions are simply treatment edema or sometimes angioneurotic edema, which can lead to severe and disfiguring swelling (**Fig. 17**). Patients who have these reactions are treated with heat and tapering steroids. True granulomatous reactions infrequently are seen and can be delayed. These may respond spontaneously but sometimes require steroid injection or surgical excision.

Nerve Injuries and Treatment in Facial Cosmetic Surgery

Babak Azizzadeh, MD, FACS[a],*, Grigoriy Mashkevich, MD[b]

KEYWORDS

• Nerve injury • Treatment • Cosmetic surgery • Face

Surgical intervention remains a popular choice in patients seeking facial rejuvenation. Although uncommon, temporary or permanent peripheral nerve injury may complicate almost any type of invasive aesthetic procedure of the face, resulting in functional and psychological consequences for patients. Prompt recognition and appropriate intervention are necessary to avoid the long-term sequelae and improve the chances of complete neurologic recovery. Depending on the type of injury, various interventions may range from observation and close follow-up to interposition nerve grafting. This article reviews the pertinent anatomy of nerves at risk in facial cosmetic surgery and discusses various management strategies for inadvertent injury to peripheral nerves of the face.

NERVES AT RISK IN FACIAL COSMETIC SURGERY: ANATOMY AND SITES OF INJURY
Motor Nerves

The dominant motor nerve to the face is the facial nerve (cranial nerve VII), which is present throughout the region targeted by almost all cosmetic procedures of the face. Therefore, a thorough understanding of its anatomy is of paramount importance in preventing injury to this critical structure.

The facial nerve, at its exit from the stylomastoid foramen, penetrates the substance of the parotid gland, by which it is well protected in the preauricular region. Within the gland, it divides into five major branches, which exit the periphery of the gland deep to the superficial muscular aponeurotic system (SMAS). Anterior to the parotid gland, distal facial nerve branches (zygomatic and buccal) are situated even deeper, under the masseteric fascia. This anatomic relationship creates a surgical plane between SMAS and the masseteric fascia, allowing for a sub-SMAS (or *deep plane*) dissection anterior to the parotid gland. As zygomatic and buccal nerves course to innervate their target midfacial muscles from underneath (zygomaticus major and minor, levator labii, and superioris alaeque nasi), a sub-SMAS plane of dissection can be followed until the first midfacial muscle is encountered (zygomaticus major), at which point the dissection must proceed superficial to this muscle (and SMAS).

Dissection in this area places zygomatic and buccal branches at risk for injury, because of their proximity. Similarly, a subperiosteal midface dissection (when performed for a midface lift) makes these deep branches vulnerable while lifting the periosteum from the anterior surface of the maxilla. Great care must be taken if performing these surgical approaches, and the use of cautery and forceful retraction should be avoided. Fortunately, anterior facial nerve branches substantially intercommunicate and innervate midfacial musculature with some redundancy. Therefore, single-branch injuries are unlikely to cause significant dysfunction of the midface.

The temporal branch of the facial nerve exits the superior aspect of the parotid gland, deep to SMAS, and crosses the zygomatic arch at the junction of the anterior one third and posterior

a Division of Head & Neck Surgery, David Geffen School of Medicine at UCLA, Los Angeles, CA, USA
b Division of Facial Plastic Surgery, Department of Otolaryngology, New York Eye & Ear Infirmary, New York, NY, USA
* Corresponding author. The Center for Facial & Nasal Plastic Surgery, 8670 Wilshire Boulevard, Suite 200, Beverly Hills, CA 90211.
E-mail address: md@facialplastics.info (B. Azizzadeh).

Oral Maxillofacial Surg Clin N Am 21 (2009) 23–29
doi:10.1016/j.coms.2008.10.003
1042-3699/08/$ – see front matter © 2009 Elsevier Inc. All rights reserved.

two thirds. Additional surface landmarks may be used to approximate the course of the temporal branch. Pitanguy's line runs from 0.5 cm inferior to the tragus to 1.5 cm above the lateral eyebrow. This location may be somewhat variable because the lateral aspect of the eyebrow is not always a precise landmark in some patients. A more consistent approximation is the line that begins at the inferior aspect of the ear lobule and bisects another line connecting the tragus and lateral canthus (**Fig. 1**).

Above the zygoma, the temporal branch enters a more superficial layer of the temporoparietal fascia and courses to innervate the superior orbicularis and frontalis muscles. Secondary to this anatomic transition, surgical lifting of the forehead, temple, and midface must be performed in a plane deep to the temporoparietal fascia. However, a face-lift dissection carried over the zygoma must be in the subcutaneous plane, which is superficial to SMAS (where the temporal branch is transitioning to the temporoparietal fascia).

The marginal branch of the facial nerve exits from the inferior aspect of the parotid gland, at the angle of the mandible, and descends up to 2 cm inferior to the body of the mandible before returning to innervate the mentalis and depressor anguli oris muscles. As these muscles are superficial to the platysma, the marginal nerve penetrates through the platysma in this region, and becomes susceptible to injury in superficial procedures such as liposuction of the jowl region. During face and neck lifting, dissection deep to platysma in the neck, or sub-SMAS dissection inferior to the border of the mandible, places the marginal nerve at risk for injury.

The spinal accessory nerve (cranial nerve XI) may be encountered during a neck lift if dissection is carried sufficiently inferior along the sternocleidomastoid muscle (SCM). This nerve crosses the SCM approximately 1 cm superior to Erb's point (location along the posterior border of SCM at which the greater auricular nerve becomes superficial). Deep dissection over the SCM should be avoided because it can lead to spinal accessory nerve palsy. Clinically, this injury manifests as a potentially debilitating shoulder dysfunction, trapezius wasting, and dull pain in the shoulder region.

Sensory Nerves

Several sensory nerves are consistently encountered during commonly performed cosmetic procedures of the face and neck. These nerves include the greater auricular, lesser occipital, infraorbital, mental, zygomaticotemporal, and zygomaticofacial nerves.

Several external landmarks are available to localize the greater auricular nerve along the posterior border of the SCM. It runs 0.5 to 1 cm parallel and posterior to the external jugular vein, and is approximately 6.5 cm inferior to the external auditory meatus. In this location over the SCM, platysma fibers become attenuated with little overlying subcutaneous tissue. Identification is further complicated by the fusion of the superficial and deep cervical fascias in this region. Thus, no surgical plane exists in this area, necessitating a sharp elevation of skin along SCM. Therefore, great care must be taken to remain superficial to avoid the greater auricular nerve injury. Another pitfall lies in the placement of sutures for suspension of SMAS to the mastoid periosteum. If placed sufficiently inferior or under undue tension, this may result in a compressive injury of the greater auricular nerve and loss of sensation over the inferior aspect of the auricle.

The lesser occipital nerve runs parallel and approximately 1 cm posterior to the greater auricular nerve, providing sensation to the superior and posterior aspects of the ear. This nerve is vulnerable to injury for the same reasons as is the greater auricular nerve.

Trigeminal nerve branches (infraorbital and mental) exit through respective foramina in the maxilla and mandible, and typically become susceptible to injury during subperiosteal dissection of the midface (midface lift, implant placement)

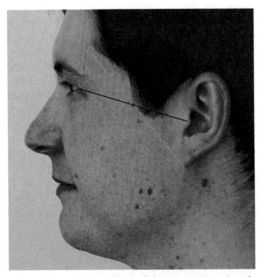

Fig. 1. External landmarks useful in approximating the course of the temporal division of the facial nerve. Blue line connects the tragus with the lateral canthus. Red point represents the midpoint of the blue line. Green line (temporal branch) bisects the blue line and runs from the inferior aspect of the lobule.

or mandible (chin implant pocket creation). These nerves, although large in caliber, are susceptible to stretch injury or transection during a subperiosteal dissection.

Zygomaticofacial and zygomaticotemporal nerves penetrate through the lateral surface of the zygomatic arch and innervate the lateral cheek and temple. Subperiosteal dissection over the zygomatic arch, as performed during the midface lift, may damage these sensory nerves and lead to a sensory deficit in the area of their distribution.

COSMETIC FACIAL PROCEDURES AND ASSOCIATED NERVE INJURIES

Several surgical approaches are currently used in facial cosmetic surgery, and therefore nerve injuries tend to be specific to the approach favored by the surgeon. Depending on the anatomic region targeted by the specific procedure, select motor and sensory nerves can become susceptible to injury. Relationships between the surgical approach and nerve injuries, and associated clinical manifestations, are listed in **Table 1**.

RATES OF NERVE INJURY IN FACIAL COSMETIC SURGERY

Several series in literature document complications of facial cosmetic surgery and report on rates of nerve injury. Most of the reviews are retrospective and may underestimate the true rate of nerve paresis and paralysis for several reasons. First, complete neurologic examinations are likely not

Table 1
Facial cosmetic procedures, associated nerves at risk, and clinical manifestations of nerve injury

	Cosmetic Facial Operation	Nerves at Risk	Clinical Manifestations
Forehead and brow	Endoscopic, trichophytic, pretrichial, or coronal brow lifts	*Motor:* Frontotemporal division of the facial nerve *Sensory:* Supraorbital and supratrochlear nerves	*Motor:* Ipsilateral forehead paresis or paralysis, with resultant brow ptosis *Sensory:* Deficit in the forehead distribution
	Direct brow lift	*Motor:* None *Sensory:* Supraorbital, supratrochlear	*Motor:* None *Sensory:* Deficit in the forehead distribution
Midface	Subperiosteal midface lift, midfacial malar or submalar augmentation (implants)	*Motor:* Zygomatic and buccal branches of the facial nerve *Sensory:* Zygomaticotemporal, zygomaticofacial, infraorbital nerves	*Motor:* Incomplete eye closure, external nasal valve collapse (nasal obstruction), drooping of the mouth corner, asymmetric smile, food spillage *Sensory:* Hyposthesia or numbness of the temporal, lateral facial, or midfacial regions
	Face lift	*Motor:* All branches of the facial nerve *Sensory:* Greater auricular, lesser occipital nerves	*Motor:* Paresis or paralysis of any portion of the face *Sensory:* Hyposthesia or numbness of the ear, inferiorly and/or superiorly
Face and neck	Chin implant	*Motor:* Marginal branch of the facial nerve *Sensory:* Mental nerve	*Motor:* Depressor anguli muscle paresis or paralysis, with resultant asymmetric smile. *Sensory:* Lower lip and chin hyposthesia or numbness
	Neck liposuction	*Motor:* Marginal branch of the facial nerve *Sensory:* None	*Motor:* Depressor labii inferioris muscle paresis or paralysis, with resultant asymmetric smile *Sensory:* None

performed routinely in busy clinical practices. Also, although motor deficits may be obvious during the interaction with the patient (and documented), sensory assessment requires a thorough physical examination and is probably not routinely performed. In addition, sensory deficits of the head and neck, although bothersome in the beginning, are generally well tolerated long-term and usually are not the primary source of patient complaints. Second, motor dysfunction, especially in the midface region, may be difficult to assess because of postoperative swelling and redundancy of innervation. Third, large reports usually originate from high-volume practices and therefore probably represent the lowest end of the spectrum for nerve injuries, simply from the experience standpoint. Therefore, published numbers reported in this article should be interpreted with caution.

During rhytidectomy, the greater auricular nerve is the most commonly injured sensory structure (1%–7%), whereas injury to the motor nerve injury occurs in approximately 2.6% of cases.[1] Depending on the series, either the marginal or temporal branches of the facial nerve seem to sustain the highest rate of motor injury. This finding has been partially explained by the lack of anastomotic and intercommunicating branches, which are present in zygomatic and buccal nerves.

Several large rhytidectomy series focusing on complications and outcomes have been reported in the literature and are briefly reviewed here. For the endoscopic brow lift, Jones and Grover[2] reported a single case of frontal branch paresis in 538 patients (0.19%), whereas Sabini and colleagues[3] found eight cases of paresis in 350 patients undergoing a combined endoscopic forehead and midface lifts (2.29%). For face-lifts, Kamer[4] presented a series of 100 deep plane rhytidectomies, with no reported events of paresis or paralysis (0%). In SMAS-platysma lifts, Daane and Owsley[5] documented cervical branch injuries in 34 of 2002 cases (1.7%). This injury was labeled a "pseudoparalysis of the marginal mandibular nerve" and full recovery in all cases occurred within 6 months. Tanna and Lindsey[6] reported no cases of nerve injury in "short scar rhytidectomy with SMAS suspension" in 1000 cases (0%). In another SMAS series of 96 patients, Sullivan and colleagues[7] documented temporary facial nerve weakness in 3% and permanent ear numbness in 1% of cases. Although these large series document the overall low rate of nerve injuries during rhytidectomy, Baker and Conley[8] noted that although facial nerve injury occurs in "less than one percent of the cases," approximately 20% of these injuries fail to undergo spontaneous return of function.

Injury to the spinal accessory nerve has also been documented during rhytidectomy.[9] Although this is highly unusual in cosmetic surgery of the neck, one should be cognizant of the nerve's location if this operation is undertaken.

PERIPHERAL NERVE ANATOMY AND CLASSIFICATION OF INJURY

Peripheral nerves contain numerous nerve fibers, which are separated by layers of connective tissue sheaths. The endoneurium envelopes individual nerve fibers, perineurium wraps around multiple nerve fibers (creating nerve fascicles), and epineurium covers the entire nerve bundle (**Fig. 2**). Mechanisms of nerve injury may be numerous and include direct trauma from anesthetic infiltration, surgical dissection, liposuction, suture placement, and use of electrocautery. Indirect trauma, such as traction injury, may also cause fiber disruption and edema within the nerve.

In 1968, Sunderland[10] published a classification system for peripheral nerve injury based on the severity of nerve disruption (**Table 2**). In this system, the most benign form of injury is neuropraxia (grade I), in which a local conduction block is present (from nerve compression or ischemia) without disruption of axoplasmic continuity. These nerves may continue to transmit the electrical signal beyond the site of the block and completely recover their function once the block is removed. This nerve injury is the only type in which distal Wallerian degeneration does not occur.

In more significant nerve injuries, axoplasmic (axonotmesis, grade II) or a neural tubule (neurotmesis, grade III) disruption leads to a Wallerian degeneration of the nerve distal to the site of injury. Axonotmesis undergoes excellent functional recovery, secondary to axonal regeneration through intact neural tubules. In contrast, neural

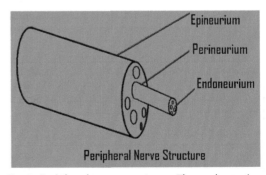

Fig. 2. Peripheral nerve anatomy. The endoneurium envelopes individual nerve fibers, perineurium wraps around multiple nerve fibers (creating nerve fascicles), and epineurium covers the entire nerve bundle.

Table 2
Sunderland classification of nerve injuries and anticipated clinical recovery

Sunderland Classification	Anatomic Injury	Clinical Manifestation and Recovery
I (neuropraxia)	Local conduction block, with preservation of axoplasmic continuity	Clinical recovery usually complete in several weeks
II (axonotmesis)	Axoplasmic disruption, endoneurium intact, with preservation of nerve sheath continuity	Wallerian degeneration, with 1 mm/d regrowth, good to excellent recovery of function
III (neurotmesis)	Endoneurium disruption, with preservation of nerve sheath continuity	Wallerian degeneration, worse degree of recovery, with synkinesis
IV (perineurium disruption)	Nerve sheath continuity preserved with intact epineurium	Wallerian degeneration, poor recovery with significant synkinesis
V (epineurium disruption)	Complete nerve transection	Paralysis

tubule disruption promotes aberrant regeneration of nerve fibers within fascicles, potentially resulting in synkinesis.

Grades IV (perineurium disruption, nerve sheath continuity preserved) and V (epineurium, or complete nerve transection) injuries confer the worst prognosis for functional recovery, because neural regeneration is severely hampered by intraneural scarring and aberrant pathway selection. Theoretically, grade V injuries do not recover any function without anatomic reapproximation of the cut ends of the nerve.

TREATMENT OF NERVE INJURIES
Preserved Nerve Continuity

Most cases of postoperative nerve dysfunction occur when little doubt exists about nerve integrity. These typically recover well with conservative management alone. Patients must be counseled that recovery is anticipated, but that it may take some time. In the immediate postoperative period, motor branch paralysis often occurs secondary to local anesthesia, which wears off within several hours and warrants no additional intervention. For nerves that sustain direct injury (eg, from traction, cautery), a typical timeframe for recovery may be anywhere from several weeks to 6 months. This timing is consistent with hat required to undergo complete Wallerian degeneration and regrowth of nerve fibers at a rate of approximately 1 mm per day.

Although intriguing from the anti-inflammatory standpoint, the role of steroids in hastening the functional recovery of nerves remains unclear. To the authors' knowledge, no studies of steroid administration have been performed in a setting of cosmetic facial surgery. However, steroids have been evaluated in other clinical scenarios involving the facial nerve, but these reports unfortunately offer conflicting recommendations.

The strongest evidence against the use of postoperative steroids for facial nerve dysfunction is based on a prospective randomized trial of patients undergoing parotid surgery.[11] The study group receiving perioperative dexamethasone derived no benefit and, in fact, displayed a median time of 150 days to recovery, compared with only 60 days in the control group. This finding is in contrast to studies documenting a beneficial impact of steroids in patients who had Bell's palsy.[12]

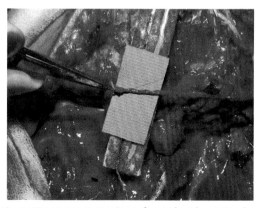

Fig. 3. Nerve anastomosis performed with a 9-0 nylon suture (fine black strand in the photograph) spanning the epineurial layer of cut ends. Typically, 3 to 4 sutures are necessary to achieve stable closure. Nerve approximation must be performed under microscope magnification and without tension.

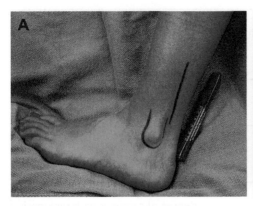
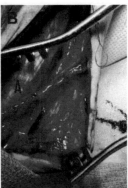

Fig. 4. Sural nerve graft. (*A*) External marking on the left lower extremity before nerve harvest. The incision is placed approximately 2 cm posterior to the lateral malleolus of the fibula, and taken superiorly as necessary to obtain sufficient graft length. This nerve can also be harvested through a stab incision with a nerve stripper. (*B*) Internal anatomy. Note the close relationship of the nerve to the vein, and a distal branching pattern, suitable in caliber to peripheral facial nerve branches. The asterisk represents the lesser saphenous vein and the arrow the sural nerve. A, Achilles tendon.

Nerve Transection Injuries

If nerve injury is confirmed intraoperatively, immediate repair should be attempted with direct anastomosis of the cut ends. Tensionless technique represents a critical aspect of any nerve repair; otherwise, regeneration of fibers may be compromised through the site of nerve coaptation. Both ends of the nerve should be freshly cut and three to four epineurial 9-0 nylon stitches be placed circumferentially to achieve an effective anastomosis (**Fig. 3**).

Nerve grafting may be required in cases where tensionless closure is not possible or in those in which nerve transection spans a segment. For facial nerve grafting, sacrificing a regional sensory nerve, such as the greater auricular, is unreasonable; sural and lateral antebrachial cutaneous nerves represent alternative sources for nerve grafting (**Fig. 4**).

Postoperative Management of Poorly Recovered or Paralytic Facial Nerve Branches

Poor recovery of the facial nerve may result in uncoordinated movement of affected muscle groups or complete paralysis. For the correction of facial synkinesis or asymmetry, botulinum toxin has been documented in several studies to be highly effective.[13,14] In cases of paralysis, the approach should be site-specific (ie, upper, middle, and lower face should be considered separately). For instance, marginal nerve paralysis may be treated with the contralateral botulinum toxin injection, depressor labii inferioris myectomy, or selective contralateral marginal mandibular neurectomy.[15–17]

SUMMARY

Several motor and sensory nerves are at risk during facial rejuvenation surgery. A thorough understanding of nerve anatomy is critical in avoiding neurologic injury, which may be severely debilitating for patients. In the event of injury, management depends on the degree of nerve disruption and may range from simple observation to exploration and grafting. Meticulous dissection technique, guided by knowledge of facial anatomy, should prevent most neurologic sequelae during facial cosmetic surgery.

REFERENCES

1. Baker SR. Rhytidectomy. In: Cummings CW, editor. Otolaryngology head & neck surgery. 4th edition. Philadelphia: Elsevier; 2005.
2. Jones BM, Grover R. Endoscopic brow lift: a personal review of 538 patients and comparison of fixation techniques. Plast Reconstr Surg 2004; 113(4):1242–50.
3. Sabini P, Wayne I, Quatela VC. Anatomical guides to precisely localize the frontal branch of the facial nerve. Arch Facial Plast Surg 2003;5:150–2.
4. Kamer FM. One hundred consecutive deep plane face-lifts. Arch Otolaryngol Head Neck Surg 1996; 122(1):17–22.
5. Daane SP, Owsley JQ. Incidence of cervical branch injury with "marginal mandibular nerve pseudoparalysis" in patients undergoing face lift. Plat Reconstr Surg 2003;111(7):2414–8.
6. Tanna N, Lindsey WH. Review of 1,000 consecutive short-scar rhytidectomies. Dermatol Surg 2008; 34(2):196–202.
7. Sullivan CA, Masin J, Maniglia AJ, et al. Complications of rhytidectomy in an otolaryngology training program. Laryngoscope 1999;109(2):198–203.
8. Baker DC, Conley J. Avoiding facial nerve injuries in rhytidectomy. Anatomical variations and pitfalls. Plast Reconstr Surg 1979;64(6):781–95.

9. Blackwell KE, Landman MD, Calcaterra TC. Spinal accessory nerve palsy: an unusual complication of rhytidectomy. Head Neck 1994;16(2):181–5.

10. Sunderland S. Nerve and nerve injuries. 2nd edition. Edinburgh: E & S Livingstone Ltd; 1968:31–60, 263–73.

11. Lee KJ, Fee WE, Terris DJ. The efficacy of corticosteroids in postparotidectomy facial nerve paresis. Laryngoscope 2002;112(11):1958–63.

12. Austin JR, Peskind SP, Austin SG, et al. Idiopathic facial nerve paralysis: a randomized double blind controlled study of placebo versus prednisone. Laryngoscope 1993;103(12):1326–33.

13. Benedetto AV. Asymmetrical smiles corrected by botulinum toxin serotype A. Dermatol Surg 2007; 33(1):S32–6.

14. De Maio M, Bento RF. Botulinum toxin in facial palsy: an effective treatment for contralateral hyperkinesis. Plast Reconstr Surg 2007;120(4):917–27.

15. Chen CK, Tang YB. Myectomy and botulinum toxin for paralysis of the marginal mandibular branch of the facial nerve: a series of 76 cases. Plast Reconstr Surg 2007;120(7):1859–64.

16. Breslow GD, Cabiling D, Kanchwala S, et al. Selective marginal mandibular neurectomy for treatment of marginal mandibular lip deformity in patients with chronic unilateral facial palsies. Plast Reconstr Surg 2005;116(5):1223–32.

17. Hussain G, Manktelow RT, Tomat LR. Depressor labii inferioris resection: an effective treatment for marginal mandibular nerve paralysis. Br J Plast Surg 2004;57(6):502–10.

How to Avoid Blepharoplasty Complications

Morris E. Hartstein, MD, FACS[a],*, Don Kikkawa, MD[b]

KEYWORDS

- Blepharoplasty • Complication • Evaluation
- Transconjunctival • Lid crease • Retraction

An unknown wise surgeon once said, "if you don't want complications, then don't operate." Complications unfortunately are part of blepharoplasty surgery. The goal of this article is to help guide the surgeon through the thought process of the preoperative evaluation, surgical planning, and actual surgery to avoid complications. With better understanding of the goals of blepharoplasty and the areas for potential problems, we hope to reduce the possibility of developing complications. As such, it is useful to divide blepharoplasty complications into the following categories:

1. Sight-threatening
2. Non–sight-threatening
   A. Problems with preoperative evaluation
      1. Functional issues (dry eye, ptosis, blepharitis, and so forth)
      2. Cosmetic issues (unrecognized brow ptosis, prolapsed lacrimal gland, and so forth)
      3. Offering the wrong operation for the problem (same operation for every patient, and so forth)
   B. Problems with surgical judgment
      1. Correct technique, poor judgment (too much skin/fat/muscle removed, brows lifted too high, and so forth)
   C. Problems with surgical technique
      1. Correct technique, performed poorly (damage to levator, asymmetric lid creases, residual fat, damage/rounding of lateral canthus, and so forth)

D. What in the world happened—unforeseen complications despite everything being done correctly

We have found if we start thinking about complications in these terms, it is easier to figure out where we went wrong and thus easier to correct the problems. The best way to avoid these complications is to think everything through clearly from the beginning. Instead of presenting a laundry list of complications and their management—but keeping them in mind—we prefer to present our preoperative and surgical approach to blepharoplasty.

VISION-THREATENING COMPLICATIONS: ORBITAL HEMORRHAGE

The preoperative history should determine whether the patient is taking any medications that could cause excessive bleeding or if the patient has a tendency to bleed. The list of medications and vitamin supplements that can lead to bleeding seems to grow longer each day. Patients should be given a list of medications and supplements to look at or be asked specifically by name what they are taking—patients may not always consider a supplement or even aspirin as a medication. Also, more patients are now on anticoagulation and for a longer period of time. For instance, patients now take Plavix for 12 months after having cardiac stents placed. Close consultation with the primary care physician

Supported in part by an unrestricted grant from Research to Prevent Blindness Foundation.
[a] Saint Louis University Eye Institute, Ophthalmology, Saint Louis University School of Medicine, 1755 South Grand Boulevard, St. Louis, MO 63104, USA
[b] Shiley Eye Center, Ophthalmology, University of California, San Diego, CA, USA
* Corresponding author.
E-mail address: mhartstein@earthlink.net (M.E. Hartstein).

Oral Maxillofacial Surg Clin N Am 21 (2009) 31–41
doi:10.1016/j.coms.2008.10.006
1042-3699/08/$ – see front matter © 2009 Elsevier Inc. All rights reserved.

is recommended. It may be best to not operate on certain patients who cannot stop their medications or for whom stopping medication would put them at greater risk for an embolic event. One must carefully weigh the risks with the patient and the primary care physician of stopping anticoagulation (embolus) versus continuing anticoagulation (hemorrhage), because there are currently no clear guidelines in this evolving area.

Bleeding during blepharoplasty surgery can come from orbicularis bleeding or from vessels within the fat pockets. Meticulous hemostasis is a given before wound closure to avoid a postoperative bleed. Postoperative bleeding may result in a hematoma or a retrobulbar hemorrhage. Smokers may be more prone to hematoma from coughing fits. Retrobulbar hemorrhage after blepharoplasty is a true emergency and if left untreated can lead to permanent blindness or decreased vision (**Fig. 1**). Clinically, there is periorbital ecchymosis, diffuse subconjunctival hemorrhage, and a tense and tight orbit. Vision may be significantly decreased and intraocular pressure elevated. This emergency should be treated immediately. The wounds should be opened and explored to see if there is a bleeding vessel. If this maneuver is not sufficient, then a lateral canthotomy and cantholysis should be performed (**Fig. 2**). Hyperosmotic agents or carbonic anhydrase inhibitors can be administered to help reduce intraocular pressure and to help restore blood flow. In rare cases of orbital hemorrhage, bony orbital decompression needs to be performed.

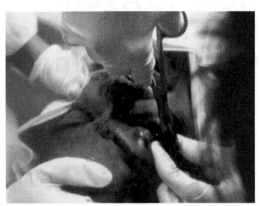

Fig. 2. Emergent lateral canthotomy for orbital hemorrhage. The key is to release the inferior crus of the lateral canthal tendon.

Meticulous hemostasis and monitoring are key to preventing a postoperative retrobulbar hemorrhage. Any evidence of severe pain, decreased vision, or significant swelling likely caused by a tense orbit should be promptly examined and not put off until the next day.[1]

NON–SIGHT-THREATENING COMPLICATIONS

All blepharoplasty patients are not the same and each should be evaluated and treated according to their individual findings. When evaluating a patient for upper blepharoplasty, we go through the following anatomic checklist (preoperative examination checklist for upper blepharoplasty; Philip L. Custer, MD, St. Louis, MO, personal communication, 2008).

Brows

Brow ptosis can contribute to dermatochalasis and fullness of the superior sulcus. Conversely, brow elevation can be a compensatory response to eyelid ptosis or dermatochalasis that diminishes the appearance of dermatochalasis. Most patients have some degree of brow asymmetry and this should be demonstrated to them during preoperative discussion. Because brow hair may have been plucked, waxed, or shaved, the natural location of the brow can be identified by palpating the brow fat pad and noting the sharp transition between the thicker brow and thinner eyelid tissue.

Bony Orbits

There can be significant individual variation in orbital size. Orbital asymmetry can also be present. A smaller orbit results in crowding and fullness of the superior sulcus, whereas patients who have larger orbits usually have a deeper and more

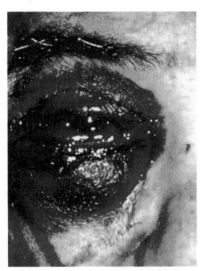

Fig. 1. Orbital hemorrhage after blepharoplasty causing a tight orbit and potentially severe visual loss. The first step is prompt diagnosis, followed by opening of the incisions.

hollow superior sulcus. The eyelid crease can be affected also and is often lower in patients who have smaller orbits. A patient who has a smaller orbit may not achieve the same surgical results as a patient who has a larger orbit, and this should be discussed preoperatively.

Eyelid Skin

Grade the amount and quality of the eyelid skin in each eyelid. Although dependent edema can sometimes develop within marked dermatochalasis, the presence of lid swelling should warrant further preoperative evaluation for conditions such as thyroid disease. Eyelid inflammation (blepharitis) can be caused by allergy, mechanical trauma, and various dermatologic conditions. Blepharitis and meibomitis can be exacerbated by surgery and should be treated before considering surgery.

Orbital Fat

The prominence and location of the fat pockets is graded before surgery. Fullness in the central or medial upper eyelid is usually related to prolapse of the orbital fat.

Lacrimal Glands

The primary lacrimal glands are located in the superolateral orbits. These glands occasionally become ptotic, contributing to fullness in the lateral upper lids.

Lid Margin

Although there is much variability, the natural position of the upper eyelid margins is usually about 2 mm below the superior corneal limbus with the patient in primary gaze. The lid margins are evaluated for symmetry, ptosis, or retraction. Further evaluation and preoperative counseling is needed if these findings are present. Review of old photographs is helpful in determining if changes are of recent onset. Blepharoplasty alone should not be considered as a way to change the position of the eyelid margin, but may be combined with ptosis repair. The lower eyelid positions are also evaluated. Preexisting lower lid retraction or scleral show can predispose a patient to complications, such as dry eye, following upper lid surgery.

Ocular Evaluation

Patients considering blepharoplasty should have an eye examination to determine if there are ocular conditions that could complicate surgery. Post-blepharoplasty dry eye can range from being a mild inconvenience to having catastrophic consequences. To evaluate a patient for dry eye, pay specific attention to the following questions:

> Does the patient currently use artificial tears?
> Do their eyes burn or have foreign body sensation?
> Do they have ocular allergies?
> Do they have systemic diseases that may be associated with dry eye, such as rheumatoid arthritis, Sjögren syndrome, or perimenopause?
> Have they had Bell palsy or prior eyelid surgery?

Prior LASIK patients may be at particularly high risk because they have an anesthetic cornea. We generally recommend waiting at least 6 months after LASIK before proceeding with blepharoplasty. Careful attention should be given to evaluating the tear film, tear evaporation, eyelid closure, and blink. Schirmer testing measures the basal tear secretion. Although the reliability of Schirmer testing may be controversial, it can help identify those patients who have severe dry eyes. A quicker and easier test is the Zone Quick Phenol Red (FCI Ophthalmics), wherein threads are placed in the inferior fornix (without anesthetic) for 15 seconds.

Visual Fields

Visual field evaluation should be performed with and without elevating the redundant eyelid tissue in patients desiring functional upper eyelid blepharoplasty. It is best to request prior determination of coverage in such individuals. The surgeon should also determine if the patient is truly seeking a functional correction or also has cosmetic motivation for the surgery. Cosmetic patients may present with functional concerns and functional patients may also have cosmetic concerns.

Photographs

External photographs are obtained to document the preoperative findings. Photos should include eyebox view, including both lateral canthi, from just above the brows down to the nasal tip, three-quarter views on each side, and full-face views, and should have proper lighting and shadowing.

Informed Consent

The risks of surgery are discussed and documented. It is reasonable to cover noticeable scarring, bleeding, infection, loss of vision, incomplete eyelid closure with ocular irritation, asymmetry, and need for additional treatment. This last point is especially important in cosmetic blepharoplasty in which minor revisions are not uncommon. Many unhappy blepharoplasty patients feel they were not warned preoperatively of potential complications or assumed the surgery was a much simpler procedure.

There are some conditions that may put patients at a higher risk than usual for complications following blepharoplasty or require specialized surgical techniques: unrealistic expectations, prior eyelid/facial surgery, dry eye symptoms, thyroid disease, prominent eyes, marked orbital asymmetry, or significant coexisting medical problems. The best way to manage complications is not to have them. By a thorough review of this preoperative checklist on each patient before surgery, many potential surgical complications can be avoided.

UPPER EYELID BLEPHAROPLASTY
Skin Marking

Skin marking is probably one of the most important steps for ensuring a successful operation so it is important to pay attention to detail (Cat Burkat, MD, Madison, WI, personal communication, 2008). Placement of the skin incision is crucial—postoperatively the eyelid crease is one of the more prominent features of the upper lid. It is helpful to mark the incisions with a fine-tip marking pen (eg, Devon #61, or Cardinal Health) before injection of local anesthetic to avoid distortion of the tissues from the anesthetic. Thicker markers spread more, especially if the lid gets wet from injection or if the eyelid opens during marking. Marker spread can lead to the lines being millimeters off, which in the cosmetic population makes a difference. Alternatively, one can prep first, then mark, inject, and score the incisions so they do not become distorted. When both sides are scored, no matter what happens to the lid the incisions will be equal. The downside is less time for hemostasis from injection, which can be compensated for by waiting or doing lower lids if scheduled (Guy G. Massry, MD, Santa Monica, CA, personal communication, 2008).

Use the existing creases, if present, and if they are symmetric and appropriate for gender. Creases can often be asymmetric, contain double lines, or be discontinuous. In addition, care must be taken if involutional ptosis is also present, because the eyelid crease may be anatomically elevated up to heights of 15 to 20 mm (due to dehiscence of the anterior fibers of the levator aponeurosis that attach to dermis and skin at the level of the lid crease). Placement of the incision at these elevated crease levels would result in

a suboptimal and unnatural appearance to the eyelids (Cat Burkat, MD, Madison, WI, personal communication, 2008). If there is no crease to use as a guide, then mark the crease as follows: 8 to 11 mm for women, 6 to 8 mm for men, with the crease incision rounder and more arched in women, and flatter and lower in men. In Asian eyelids, the medial aspects of the markings should blend into the epicanthal fold. In addition, the height of the eyelid crease in Asians is much lower, at 4 to 6 mm. Placing the incision at the normal 8- to 11-mm height in an Asian patient would result in a westernized eyelid that would be unfavorable to the Asian patient; most Asians desire a defined, low crease, not a high western crease.[2]

Another way to approach skin marking is to recall that the upper eyelid skin should measure about 20 mm from eyelid margin to the eyebrow skin (Cat Burkat, MD, Madison, WI, personal communication, 2008). For the beginning blepharoplasty surgeon, this measurement can help eliminate the risk for postoperative lagophthalmos from overaggressive tissue excision. One way to measure this out is as follows: Subtract the height of the eyelid crease from a total of 20 mm. This amount is then measured from the inferior edge of brow skin, which thus represents the superior border of the skin flap to be removed. When marking, care should be taken to avoid confusing the true junction of the inferior brow (where the thin eyelid skin transitions to thicker, larger porous brow skin with a different color) in women who pluck their eyebrows to a higher height. Do not measure the skin of the upper incision to the plucked eyebrow level; this may result in excessive skin removal and a harsh transition zone at the upper incision. At this point, the pinch technique can be used to confirm that an adequate 19 to 20 mm of skin is preserved. This technique is done by pinching together the skin between the inferior and superior markings and measuring the remaining skin from the eyelid margin to the brow skin. If the skin pinch results in tightness to the thin eyelid skin, vertical striae to the skin, or retraction or eversion of the eyelid margin, too much skin is being excised.

Complication: Asymmetric Eyelid Crease

A high eyelid crease is more difficult to correct than a lower eyelid crease. Also, a high crease in males is considered more undesirable because it produces a more feminine appearance (**Fig. 3**). It is easier to raise a low crease than to lower a high crease. If there are asymmetric creases, one should discuss with the patient using the higher crease as the guide. To raise a low crease,

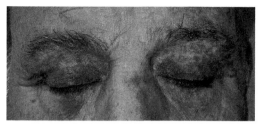

Fig. 3. Asymmetric and high creases in a male after upper blepharoplasty. To correct, it would be easier to raise the lower crease on the right.

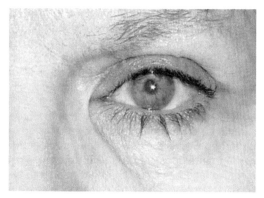

Fig. 4. Medial canthal web after upper blepharoplasty. Massage and steroid injections can help. Sometimes tissue rearrangement is needed.

an incision is made at the new desired crease level. The tissues under the old, low crease are undermined as are the pretarsal tissues, to allow them to elevate freely. Crease-forming sutures are then placed at the level of the new incision.[1] To lower a high crease, the new incision is placed beneath the old high crease. The tissues are undermined in a superior direction. To prevent re-adherence at the old crease level, it may be necessary to place a barrier, such as a thin dermis fat graft, between the septum and levator. Again, crease-forming sutures are placed in an interrupted fashion.

The medial extent of the skin marking is made no further medial than the upper punctum. Incisions that extend medial to the punctum increase the risk for webbing in the nasal eyelid region. Care should be taken not to excise too much tissue medially because this can cause webbing or lag. If there remains an excess of skin medially, the incision can be flared upward at the punctum and the same can be done laterally. Preoperatively, by pulling on the bridge of the nose, one can observe if the patient has a tendency to form a medial canthal web and thus plan and counsel the patient.

Complication: Medial Canthal Webbing

Again, the best treatment is prevention (**Fig. 4**). Intraoperatively, the nasal end of the lid crease mark should not extend past the punctum, or it should flare upward slightly after reaching the punctum. During closure, the running suture can be started just lateral to the medial-most aspect of the incision. Bites of orbicularis and the edge of levator can be incorporated to reduce tension on the medial incision, or interrupted sutures can be placed medially before starting the running suture. If a medial canthal web does result, time, massage, and steroid injections can help. If it persists, then revision by Y-V–type incisions is warranted.

The lateral extent of the incision should not extend into the thicker temporal skin. Laterally

one must balance skin excision with brow position and discuss reasonable outcomes with patients preoperatively. More aggressive excision laterally is acceptable because the patient is unlikely to develop corneal problems from excess temporal skin excision unless to the extreme. The brow tends to give and compensate for this. Unfortunately, the brow can become lowered.

In patients who express a desire for more pretarsal tarsal show laterally may require a browlift (not to elevate, but at least to stabilize brow height). Elevating the temporal brow also shortens the lateral extent of the excision by reducing the pseudo-dermatochalasis components of the full temporal lid (by eliminating brow ptosis). In addition, postoperative sub-brow Botox injections (6U per side) are helpful during recovery. Residual temporal skin excess is a common complication of upper blepharoplasty. This complication may result from inadequate excision or postoperative frontalis relaxation. It is easily corrected by excising a small ellipse of temporal skin (**Fig. 5**) (Guy G. Massry, MD, Santa Monica, CA, personal communication, 2008).

Various options are available for making the skin incision, such as the Ellman radiofrequency unit

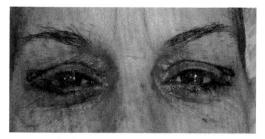

Fig. 5. Residual temporal excess after upper blepharoplasty is marked for excision and repair.

with a microdissection tip, or the monopolar unit with a Colorado tip, CO_2 laser, or a standard 15 blade. If using a 15 blade, the 15c offers a more slender blade appropriate for eyelid skin. The skin and orbicularis muscle are removed as single flaps generally, although a skin flap alone could be removed if there is preoperative concern for poor eyelid closure function. More and more, there is a trend to preserving orbicularis muscle so as not to impair eyelid closure. There is enough lid thinning (anteroposterior) by skin excision. Postoperative lagophthalmos can be divided into two types: (1) tethered, due to a skin shortage or septal scar, and (2) paretic (more common), due to orbicularis weakness. Lagophthalmos (especially nocturnal) can occur even with adequate skin, and is more likely to occur from orbicularis weakness; therefore, avoid manipulating the orbicularis as much as possible.

Next, the fat pads are addressed if they are prominent on the preoperative evaluation. The trend in upper eyelid blepharoplasty has shifted to preservation, repositioning, or filling of the upper lid fat, rather than aggressive removal. In general, limited fat removal should be performed to avoid the appearance of a hollow superior sulcus. If debulking is indicated, the fat should be conservatively removed over a curved hemostat to avoid orbital hemorrhage. Intraoperatively, only the fat that easily presents should be removed. When considering medial fat removal, bear in mind the location of the trochlea and superior oblique tendon and the numerous fibrous attachments of these structures to the orbital fat. Generally, the orbital fat pads can be thermally sculpted with the Ellman roundball tip or the Colorado tip over an intact orbital septum, which limits the risk for hemorrhage or injury to adjacent structures and requires less operative time.

Complication: Oversculpted, Deep Superior Sulcus

Preoperative evaluation is key to identifying those at risk for this problem. Overaggressive removal of the central fat pad is usually the cause (**Fig. 6**). To correct this problem, residual fat pedicles may be mobilized and advanced, or fat/filler injections may be used, placing the material juts under the superior orbital rim.

In the lateral upper eyelid, a prolapsed lacrimal gland may be found in up to 10% to 15% of young patients undergoing blepharoplasty. The lacrimal gland exhibits a characteristic whitish color and globular appearance. It is crucial to correctly identify this structure intraoperatively, because inadvertent lacrimal lobectomy may lead to

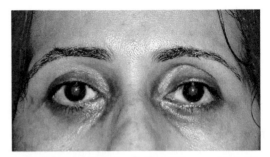

Fig. 6. Overaggressive sculpting left upper lid after blepharoplasty leads to hollow sulcus and crease deformity.

possible postoperative hemorrhage or dry eye. On the other hand, if left in a prolapsed position, this may result in eyelid asymmetry, persistent lateral fullness, and therefore poor cosmesis. The lacrimal gland can easily be resuspended under the superolateral orbit with several interrupted sutures. We perform less brow fat sculpting in recent years and, in some cases, believe more in fat injections to elevate the ptotic brow fat pad.

Closure issues

The lateral area is dynamic so locking lateral sutures (a few) during the running suture are key for support to prevent dehiscence. Another option is to place several interrupted sutures laterally and then close with a running suture. To emphasize or reform the lid crease, one can place two to three interrupted sutures, taking a bite of skin–pretarsal orbicularis–skin (**Fig. 7**). This procedure also controls exactly where the lid crease is. Some patients complain of misalignment of the relaxed skin tension lines of the lids after blepharoplasty. An arched incision with slight misalignment in patients who have obvious vertical lines can lead to this problem. Placing two cardinal sutures

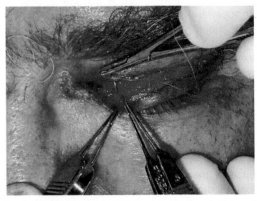

Fig. 7. Crease-forming sutures are placed through skin–levator edge (or pretarsal orbicularis)–skin.

(centrally and temporally) in the blepharoplasty incision turns a long arched incision into three small ellipses and reduces the chance of webbing and skin malalignment (Guy G. Massry, MD, Santa Monica, CA, personal communication, 2008).

Complication: Milia

Milia occur as a cystic elevation where the suture needle passed through the skin. These can be bothersome to the patient. Milia have been seen to occur with all suture types, although perhaps less with 6-0 Prolene. Subcuticular sutures and early removal may help cut down on the frequency of milia. Milia can disappear spontaneously but this can take place over several months. Some patients prefer to have them removed sooner rather than wait. Traditionally, a small needle or scissors can be used to unroof the milia.[1] Alternatively, 0.5 toothed forceps can be used effectively to impale the milia with minimal discomfort.

Complication: Wound Dehiscence

Wound dehiscence can occur after upper blepharoplasty, particularly when absorbable sutures are used. Many wound dehiscences can be managed conservatively, with just topical ointment. There may be exudates but frank infection is rare. The edges can be reapproximated and resutured but often do well healing by secondary intention.

Complication: Dog Ears

Dog ears may form at either the medial or lateral end of the incision. These can be minimized by equalizing tension across the upper eyelid incision. Careful placement of a fine hemostat (medially) and a single skin hook (laterally) enables closure of the upper blepharoplasty incision often without the need for a surgical assistant (Peter Levin, MD, Palo Alto, CA, personal communication, 2008).

Complication: Lagophthalmos and Dry Eye

The most obvious cause of post-blepharoplasty dry eye is lagophthalmos, from too much tissue removal, lower lid retraction, or both (**Fig. 8**). Dry eye may also occur in the absence of lagophthalmos. Milder cases of exposure and dry eye can be managed with massage and artificial tears. Corrective surgical procedures for lagophthalmos include: tarsorrhaphy, skin graft, spacer graft, and midface lift.[3] Another more subtle and more common cause of dry eye is a decreased blink excursion where there is no obvious lagophthalmos. Fortunately, most cases of post-blepharoplasty dry eye are transient and resolve spontaneously.

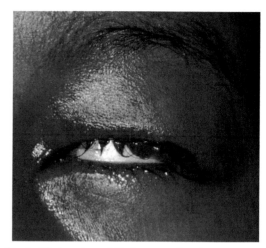

Fig. 8. Obvious lagophthalmos causing dry eye.

Supportive measures should be tailored to the specific tear film problem: deficiency in the aqueous layer is easily treated with over-the-counter artificial tear supplements. Punctal plugs (not intracanalicular) can be helpful too. Warm compresses with massage can help with meibomian gland dysfunction, which can worsen postoperatively, leading to increased tear evaporation. Products to improve meibomian gland dysfunction include doxycycline, vitamin supplements (such as Hydroeye, www.sciencebasedhealth.com) containing omega-3, cod liver oil capsules, flaxseed oil capsules, and soy supplements.

Complication: Allergy

Some patients may develop an allergic reaction to postoperative ointments, especially those containing neomycin, although it can occur with any ointment. This reaction can be distressing to the patient and to the surgeon. It is best to discontinue all topical medications. If the reaction is severe, then topical steroids can be given but we prefer only Vaseline for lubrication of the dry skin.

LOWER EYELID BLEPHAROPLASTY

We believe lower blepharoplasty is a much more complicated procedure than upper lid blepharoplasty. The preoperative evaluation is perhaps even more critical in these patients to ensure a successful operation. The cookie-cutter approach is to be discouraged in any cosmetic surgery but perhaps nowhere more so than the lower lid. There are many different factors at play in the lower lid and these must be identified and discussed thoroughly with the patient preoperatively before an appropriate surgical plan can be established. Each individual patient has specific and somewhat unique anatomic problems that require different surgical techniques to correct (Sheri L. DeMartelaere, MD, Todd R. Shepler, MD, Sean M. Blaydon, MD, Russell W. Neuhaus, MD, John W. Shore, MD, Austin, TX, personal communication, 2008).

In addition to an ocular examination as listed for upper blepharoplasty, we go through a preoperative checklist when evaluating patients for lower blepharoplasty (preoperative checklist for lower blepharoplasty, John Siddens, MD, Greenville, SC, personal communication, 2008):

- The quality and amount of excess skin is evaluated. This evaluation can be done while the patient looks straight ahead and upward. While looking upward, the lower eyelid skin is put on stretch and any excess skin with the lid in this position can be excised with less risk for producing cicatricial retraction or ectropion after lower eyelid blepharoplasty.
- Fat pockets attributable to pseudoherniation are noted by looking for areas of fullness as the patient looks straight ahead and then in upgaze. Gentle pressure can be applied to the globe through the closed upper eyelid to make these areas of fat prolapse bulge. These areas of fullness may be diminished or absent when the patient is lying supine at the time of surgery. The presence of festoons or chronic eyelid edema may indicate chronic inflammation, which may reoccur postoperatively. One should particularly note the location and amount of the lateral fat pad. This pad can be much more difficult to reach surgically. Orbicularis hypertrophy may also contribute to lower lid fullness and may need to be addressed.
- Look for lower eyelid laxity and ectropion that may need to be addressed at the time of surgery. Lower eyelid retraction should be identified preoperatively. Cause of the retraction should be determined, such as cicatricial skin changes versus poor bony support and prominence of the globe.
- Lower lid distraction test: Pull the lower eyelid away from the eye. Normally, the eyelid should not be able to be pulled more than 6 mm from the globe.
- Snap-back test: This test is performed by pulling the lower eyelid downward and observing how quickly it snaps back against the globe. If there is significant laxity, the eyelid may not snap back until the patient

blinks (**Fig. 9**A–B). If the distraction test and the snap-back test demonstrate laxity, then the patient is at risk for postoperative lid malposition and should probably have a lid-tightening procedure with the blepharoplasty.

- Another variation on this is the gape test. If the eyelid tone is normal, the lower eyelids move upward when the patient is in upgaze. Even with the mouth open, the eyelid excursion should be close to normal. If lid laxity or retraction is present, the lids do not move upward, as demonstrated with increased scleral show (a positive gape test).
- Lateral laxity: The lower eyelid at the lateral canthus can be evaluated by pulling the lateral lower eyelid toward the nose. The lateral canthus should move only minimally with this maneuver.
- Medial laxity: The medial canthal tendon can be similarly evaluated by pulling the medial lower eyelid laterally. If the lower punctum approaches the corneal limbus then there is significant medial canthal laxity. Look for punctal eversion or medial ectropion that may need to be corrected at the time of surgery.

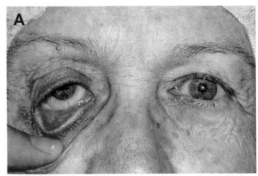

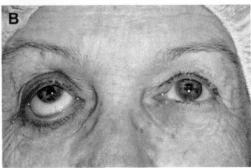

Fig. 9. (A) The snap-back test is performed by distracting the lower lid, and (B) observing if it snaps back to the globe before initiation of a blink. This patient demonstrates poor snap-back tone.

- Assess the relationship of the lower eyelid with the mid-face. Pay particular attention to the presence of suborbicularis oculi fat and malar fat pad descent or atrophy, prominent tear trough deformities, and adequate maxillary bony support of the lower eyelid and globe (Sheri L. DeMartelaere, MD, Todd R. Shepler, MD, Sean M. Blaydon, MD, Russell W. Neuhaus, MD, John W. Shore, MD, Austin, TX, personal communication, 2008).

LOWER BLEPHAROPLASTY SURGERY

After evaluating the patient, the potential layers can be addressed in the following order: fat, muscle, skin (Guy G. Massry, MD, Santa Monica, CA, personal communication, 2008). The fat is addressed first. We prefer the transconjunctival incision to a transcutaneous incision because this decreases the chance of lower lid retraction. The transconjunctival incision can be performed with a CO_2 laser, a radiofrequency unit, a monopolar tip, or even carefully with a high-temperature cautery. There has been a shift in how we address fat with a more conservative approach as opposed to just removing the fat. Our understanding of the aging process as having to do with volume loss has changed the way we approach the lower lid fat pads. Draping or repositioning fat pedicles over the inferior orbital rim is often preferable to significant fat excision (**Fig. 10**).[4] When sculpting the fat, meticulous hemostasis is critical in lower eyelid blepharoplasty. Fat can be removed/sculpted with the laser, monopolar unit, or the clamp, cut, and cautery technique using a small hemostat, Westcott scissors, and the bipolar cautery, respectively. Orbicularis muscle may be addressed by performing a strap, with or without a tarsal strip or canthopexy. If there is hypertrophic orbicularis, this can be gently debulked through a skin incision or can easily be treated with low-dose Botox injections.

If there is excessive skin laxity, skin removal can be useful if done conservatively using the pinch technique, possibly in conjunction with a horizontal tightening of the lower eyelid. The fat is still addressed through a transconjunctival incision—we rarely remove herniated fat through a transcutaneous incision. If skin pinch only is performed one can still perform retractor lysis. A transconjunctival incision is made and continued through the retractors with blunt dissection inferiorly with an applicator for 8 to 10 mm; this elevates the lid 2 to 3 mm and counteracts downward tension on the lid from a skin excision. A temporal intermarginal suture (gray line–gray line) using 5-0 chromic can be added for support. During healing whenever the upper lid opens it elevates lower lid, especially temporally where retraction is most common. The suture is left in for 1 week, which works well to decrease the complication of lid retraction (Guy G. Massry, MD, Santa Monica, CA, personal communication, 2008). Alternatively, if the patient is a CO_2 laser candidate, the lower eyelid skin can be tightened with resurfacing. Patient selection is critical because this should only be performed on the lighter skin types, and patients need to be counseled about possible persistent erythema or pigment changes.

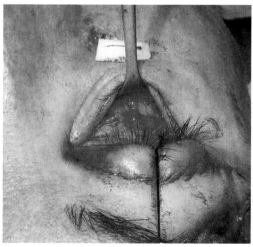

Fig. 10. Through a transconjunctival approach, fat is repositioned over the orbital rim and secured with a suture and bolster.

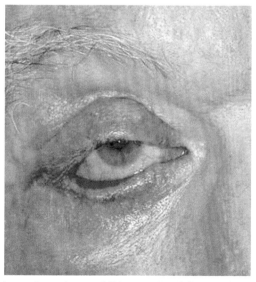

Fig. 11. Ectropion and lid retraction following lower blepharoplasty.

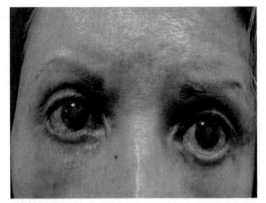

Fig. 12. Lower lid retraction, sclera show, and rounded lateral canthal angel following lower blepharoplasty.

It is important to pay attention to the lateral canthus. If there is laxity, it needs tightening or reinforcing. If there is any question as to the degree of laxity, if we are performing a trans-lid midface lift, or if it is a revision procedure, then we likely perform a full tarsal strip procedure to secure the lateral canthus.[5–9] If there is minimal laxity only, then we believe a suture canthopexy suffices, whereby a suture is placed from the inferior crus of the lateral canthal tendon to the lateral orbital rim. Patients who have negative vector eyes—prominent globes, malar ptosis, and inferior scleral show—may likely require additional support at the lateral canthus. Excessive skin removal, orienting the lateral skin too vertically, or not addressing the negative vector can all result in a rounded and downward displaced lateral canthus.

Complications

As in the upper lid, lower blepharoplasty patients can develop dry eyes, persistent edema/chemosis, allergic reactions, and so forth, and the treatment is similar to what was outlined previously. Sometimes residual fat is noted, especially laterally. It is important to make sure you clearly identify the lateral fat pad, which can often sit more anteriorly. Conversely, one of the more common complications of lower blepharoplasty is oversculpting or removal of too much fat, which eventually can give the patient a hollow or sunken look. The key to avoiding this is to be more conservative with fat removal and possibly combine the blepharoplasty surgery with a midface lift or fat/filler injections. With the increased emphasis on volumization of the lower lid/tear trough/midface area, there have been more complications. Fat injections are a wonderful adjunct to lower lid surgery, but these can also lead to a lumpy/bumpy appearance and can be difficult to remove because the fat is deposited in multiple planes. Likewise, synthetic fillers, if placed too superficially in the tear trough region, can lead to a lumpy appearance. For the beginning surgeon, the periorbital area is probably the least forgiving for fat/filler injections.

Complications: Eyelid Malposition

One of the most common and distressing complications of lower blepharoplasty is eyelid malposition. This complication can take the form of either lower lid retraction, ectropion, or both (**Fig. 11**). These complications are most often

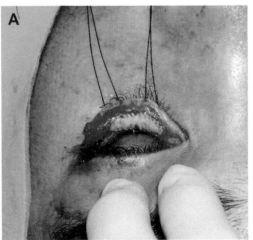
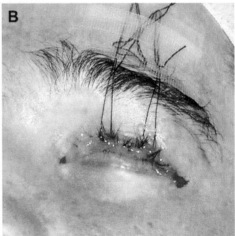

Fig. 13. (A) Repair of lower lid retraction often includes placement of a spacer graft (hard palate in this case) after scar lysis. (B) Following lower lid reconstruction, the lid is placed on upward stretch for 5 to 7 days.

associated with the transcutaneous approach. On healing the septum can contract and pull the lower lid down along with the lateral canthus, giving rise to the rounded lateral canthal angle. The patient who has postoperative lid retraction may present with sclera show, tearing, rounding of the lateral canthal angle, and the "surgical look" (**Fig. 12**).The transconjunctival route avoids violating the septum and thus has less of a chance of septal scarring causing problems. It is not just the surgical approach that can lead to this complication, however. Patients who have negative-vector eyes are more at risk for this. To determine the extent of middle lamella scarring, apply upward traction on the lid: septal scarring limits or tethers the lid on upgaze. Anterior lamellar shortage limits the lid in upgaze but the lid is mobile. Lid retraction often has components of both. If there is significant skin shortage and tether, then the treatment may include skin grafts.

Management of these cases can be challenging. For early cases with mild retraction, it may be sufficient to lyse the scar tissue and resuspend the lid with a canthoplasty. The scar tissue can be lysed transconjunctivally so as not to disturb the area of the previous skin incision. For severe or longstanding cases of lid retraction, a simple canthoplasty will not suffice and may even make matters worse. For these types of cases, surgical repair must include the following steps: lysis of the scar tissue (preferably through a virgin plane, transconjunctival approach), placement of a spacer graft (eg, hard palate, dermis fat, AlloDerm, synthetic collagen, and so forth), elevation of the midface (preferably through a subperiosteal approach with complete degloving), and lower lid traction sutures to keep the lid in an overcorrected position for 5 to 7 days. Even so, success is not guaranteed and patients should be counseled preoperatively (**Fig. 13**A,B).[10–16]

SUMMARY

Complications are an unfortunate occurrence for anyone who performs blepharoplasty surgery. We have found it helpful to group complications into the categories listed above. Thinking about how the complication arose and determining its source can help avoid it in the future. We hope readers will incorporate some of the guidelines for preoperative planning and surgery listed in this article to enhance the success rate and manage the pitfalls of cosmetic blepharoplasty.

REFERENCES

1. Putterman A, editor. Cosmetic oculoplastic surgery. London: WB Saunders; 1999.
2. Chen WPD. Asian blepharoplasty—a surgical atlas. Boston: Butterworth-Heinemann; 1994.
3. Shorr N, Goldberg RA, McCann JD, et al. Upper eyelid skin grafting: an effective treatment for lagophthalmos following blepharoplasty. Plast Reconstr Surg 2003;112(5):1444–8.
4. Mohadjer Y, Holds JB. Cosmetic lower eyelid blepharoplasty with fat repositioning via intra-SOOF dissection: surgical technique and initial outcomes. Ophthal Plast Reconstr Surg 2006;22(6):409–13.
5. Anderson RL, Gordy DD. The tarsal strip procedure. Arch Ophthalmol 1979;97(11):2192–6.
6. Jordan DR, Anderson RL. The lateral tarsal strip revisited. The enhanced tarsal strip. Arch Ophthalmol 1989;107(4):604–6.
7. Lemke BN, Sires BS, Dortzbach RK. A tarsal strip-periosteal flap technique for lateral canthal fixation. Ophthalmic Surg Lasers 1999;30(3):232–6.
8. Liu D. Lower eyelid tightening: a comparative study. Ophthal Plast Reconstr Surg 1997;13(3): 199–203.
9. Della Rocca DA. The lateral tarsal strip: illustrated pearls. Facial Plast Surg 2007;23(3):200–2.
10. Patel BC, Patipa M, Anderson RL, et al. Management of postblepharoplasty lower eyelid retraction with hard palate grafts and lateral tarsal strip. Plast Reconstr Surg 1997;99(5):1251–60.
11. Shorr N, Fallor MK. "Madame Butterfly" procedure: combined cheek and lateral canthal suspension procedure for post-blepharoplasty, "round eye," and lower eyelid retraction. Ophthal Plast Reconstr Surg 1985;1(4):229–35.
12. Sullivan SA, Dailey RA. Endoscopic subperiosteal midface lift: surgical technique with indications and outcomes. Ophthal Plast Reconstr Surg 2002; 18(5):319–30 [discussion: 329–30].
13. Wearne MJ, Sandy C, Rose GE, et al. Autogenous hard palate mucosa: the ideal lower eyelid spacer? Br J Ophthalmol 2001;85(10):1183–7.
14. Cohen MS, Shorr N. Eyelid reconstruction with hard palate mucosa grafts. Ophthal Plast Reconstr Surg 1992;8(3):183–95.
15. Li TG, Shorr N, Goldberg RA. Comparison of the efficacy of hard palate grafts with acellular human dermis grafts in lower eyelid surgery. Plast Reconstr Surg 2005;116(3):873–8 [discussion: 879–80].
16. Korn BS, Kikkawa DO, Cohen SR, et al. Treatment of lower eyelid malposition with dermis fat grafting. Ophthalmology 115(4):744–51.

Complications of Neck Liposuction and Submentoplasty

James Koehler, MD, DDS

KEYWORDS

- Liposuction • Submentoplasty • Platysma
- Laser assisted liposuction • Submandibular gland ptosis

Each year the demand for cosmetic surgery procedures has increased and many surgeons have incorporated these techniques into their practice. The biggest challenge that faces surgeons is obtaining predictable results without complications. As with any surgery, complications occur from time to time. Having the knowledge and skill to deal with these complications is paramount. As long as the surgeon has good rapport with the patient, they are given the opportunity to care properly for these unfavorable results.

Many times, patients desiring improved neck and jawline contours are looking for minimally invasive procedures and are not interested in undergoing extensive face-lifting procedures. Realizing the limitations, surgeons may offer their patient such procedures as liposuction and submentoplasty. Even though these procedures are less involved than a face-lift, still many pitfalls can occur that can result in an unfavorable result and a disappointed patient. Proper patient selection and choosing the correct operation are crucial to avoiding these situations. This article focuses on the common complications of neck liposuction and submentoplasty and reviews their management and avoidance.

PATIENT ASSESSMENT AND PROCEDURE SELECTION

After a detailed history, the initial assessment should rule out any pathologic processes that may be contributing to a poor neck and jawline, such as thyroid hyperplasia or salivary gland pathology. In the absence of pathology, the skin tone and fatty deposits of the neck should be evaluated. In general, a younger patient with good skin tone and preplatysmal fat deposits is a better candidate for liposuction. Determining the amount of preplatysmal fat can be difficult. By gently pinching the skin with the fingers one can try to estimate the amount of preplatysmal fat. In the heavy neck patient there is likely a fair amount of fat below the platysma, which cannot be treated with liposuction alone. Patients with subplatysmal fat deposits do not respond well to liposuction alone and are often left with a poor chin-neck angle and submental fullness. Provided the patient has adequate skin tone, a submentoplasty should be considered in these circumstances, because subplatysmal fat can be visualized and resected. Submentoplasty is an excellent procedure for improving neck contour in patients who have platysmal banding, subplatysmal fat deposits, and mild submental cutis laxis without significant jowling. This procedure involves a platysmaplasty and the removal of supraplatysmal and subplatysmal fat through a submental incision. Patient selection is critical to avoid complications. Both liposuction and submentoplasty procedures require that the patient have good skin tone to obtain a smooth result. Patients with significant laxity and poor tone should not be selected for these procedures and the patient should be offered some type of face-lift procedure.

Signs of an aging neck include jowling and platysmal banding. Although platysmal banding can be dramatically improved with an aggressive submentoplasty, it must be remembered that the most appropriate procedure for combined jowling and platysmal banding or laxity is often a cervicofacial rhytidectomy with or without a concurrent submentoplasty.

Tulsa Surgical Arts, 7322 East 91st Street, Tulsa, OK 74133, USA
E-mail address: james@tulsasurgicalarts.com

Oral Maxillofacial Surg Clin N Am 21 (2009) 43–52
doi:10.1016/j.coms.2008.10.008
1042-3699/08/$ – see front matter © 2009 Elsevier Inc. All rights reserved.

oralmaxsurgery.theclinics.com

To provide appropriate patient expectations, several anatomic features should be considered. If the patient has a low hyoid position as determined by neck palpation, a good neck contour may not be achievable even with a flawlessly performed surgery. Recognizing this preoperatively allows the surgeon to discuss the limitations of the procedure or alternatives, such as camouflaging with a chin implant. It is also important to evaluate the presence of large or ptotic submandibular glands preoperatively. If a patient has prominent submandibular glands, the surgeon must either address this with a partial submandibular gland resection or prepare the patient for the possibility of fullness in this area after the procedure.[1] Performing partial submandibular gland resection through a submental incision is a difficult procedure and is not recommended for those without significant experience. Complications can be higher with this procedure compared with liposuction and surgical skill and patient selection are extremely important.

Liposuction is by far one of the most popular cosmetic procedures for both men and women. Advances in liposuction include the use of tumescent solution, ultrasonic cannulae, power cannulae, and laser-assisted techniques. All surgical techniques require significant training and understanding of the limitations of the procedure. More aggressive tools, such as ultrasonic cannulae, should only be used by those experienced with liposuction. Today the trend is to use small cannulae 1 to 2 mm in diameter. The goal for cervicofacial liposuction is to resculpt the neck to improve the contour, not to remove all the fat.[2] Patients are instructed preoperatively that once fat is removed from liposuction, it is expected that the skin shrinks to take on the new contour. It is important to warn the patient that if excess skin laxity develops after the procedure, they may require additional surgical procedures.

TUMESCENT ANESTHESIA

Tumescent anesthesia originated in the dermatology literature where safe liposuction could be performed under local anesthesia alone. It was found that using a dilute solution of lidocaine and epinephrine decreased the blood loss during liposuction and provided safety to the technique.[3–5] Even though there is minimal blood loss with submental liposuction, tumescent anesthesia distends the tissue plane between the platysma and the skin and facilitates the liposuction procedure.[6]

Although the rate of absorption of lidocaine and epinephrine in the face is much faster because of the excellent blood supply, toxicity is extremely rare because of the low volume of fluid injected.

Likewise, the potential for drug interactions is also unlikely as compared with large-volume body liposuction. Serial plasma lidocaine levels have been measured when using tumescent anesthesia on the face. In one study, the peak plasma levels averaged 2.7 µg/mL and the highest level found in the series was 3.3 µg/mL. Also, the serum levels normally peaked at 1 hour after administration rather than 12 hours body tumescence.[7] Premedication with clonidine has been shown greatly to reduce the incidence of intraoperative and postoperative tachycardia with tumescent local. I typically have the patient place a 0.2-mg clonidine patch on the shoulder the morning of surgery. The patch is removed the next day.

OVERRESECTION OF FAT AND PLATYSMAL BANDS

The technique for cervicofacial liposuction has evolved over the years.[8–16] Previously, surgeons used large spatulated cannulae to extract as much fat as possible from the neck. The initial results were often good, but over time patients developed a skeletonized appearance of the neck. Once the skin has retracted and fibrosis has occurred, this can be a challenging problem to treat.

To avoid this problem it is usually best to use a small 1.5- or 2-mm microliposuction cannula. Small cannulae decrease the likelihood of having uneven or lumpy results. It is important that the cannula opening always be pointed toward the platysma. If the cannula is facing the skin, it can result in gouging of the dermal tissues and cause increased scarring, induration, and palpable skin irregularities. Ultrasonic liposuction cannulae, although available for facial liposuction, are not recommended in this region because the amount of fat is minimal and the risk of thermal injury to dermal tissues is too great unless the surgeon has significant experience with ultrasonic liposuction.

Autologous fat transfer may be needed to correct irregularities or overresection of fat. Fat grafting techniques have been extensively described. Many discussions arise as to how the fat should be treated, and this is outside the scope of this article. Keys to success involve the atraumatic harvesting of fat using 10-mL syringes attached to a small-diameter blunt cannula (1–2 mm). The abdomen usually is a good site for fat harvest through a stab incision in the umbilicus. The supranatant fat may be washed and treated and then should be transferred into 1-mL syringes and injected into multiple subdermal tunnels using a fine 16-gauge injection cannula. Some cannulae have a forked tip that allows the surgeon to break-up any subdermal adhesions and facilitate placement of the fat. Patients typically swell extensively after fat grafting and should be warned of this preoperatively. Overcorrection with grafting should be done, because not all the fat survives. The predictability of fat transfer is debatable and the patient should understand that several sessions may be required.

In some cases, the removal of fat unmasks underlying platysmal banding. If the neck contour is satisfactory, mild cases of platysmal banding can be managed by injection of botulinum toxin A into the areas of banding. Each band may require variable dosing and a typical band requires 20 units botulinum toxin A.[17] The dose should be distributed along the band with the injections sites spaced 1.5 cm apart. This needs to be repeated approximately every 4 months and may be used as a palliative treatment until more definitive treatment, such as submentoplasty with excision of platysmal bands or platysmaplasty, is performed. Caution should be taken if treatment involves excision of the platysma muscle. If there is insufficient fat on the skin flaps or the removal is not performed evenly, significant irregularities can occur and are difficult to correct with fat grafting.

Liposuction of the jowls, if performed at all, should be done conservatively. Jowling should be corrected with face-lift techniques and liposuction in this area can create a very unnatural appearance. Placing a small prejowl chin implant is an alternative to liposuctioning jowls in patients unwilling to undergo face-lift surgery. Solid silicone prejowl chin implants do not increase chin projection but do provide some fullness just anterior to the jowls thereby camouflaging the extent if jowling. The prejowl implant may add width to the chin and this should be discussed with the patient before surgery.

The so-called "cobra neck" deformity can occur with submentoplasty and usually results from overresection of subplatysmal fat in the midline of the neck. A relative deformity can also occur because of inadequate removal of fat laterally, giving the appearance of a sunken area in the submental region. Even removal of fat is essential to preventing this problem (**Fig. 1**). Leaving an adequate layer of fat on the skin flaps also helps mask minor irregularities. In patients who have decussation of the platysma at the midline, it may be necessary to release the platysma at the level of

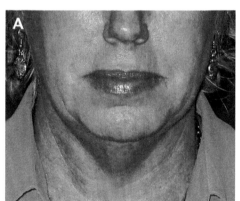
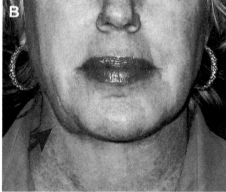
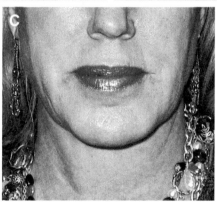

Fig.1. (*A*) Preoperative view of a 58-year-old woman with submental fullness. (*B*) The patient underwent submentoplasty but had residual fatty deposits in the right jowl and submental region (*arrow*). (*C*) The area was effectively treated with minor liposuction under local anesthesia.

the hyoid bone and advance it to the midline to provide a smooth contour to the neck. This is especially true in thinner patients with less fat deposits.

UNDIAGNOSED SUBMANDIBULAR GLAND PTOSIS

Recognizing submandibular gland enlargement or ptosis preoperatively is difficult and often overlooked before liposuction or submentoplasty procedures. Ptosis of the submandibular gland can occur with age or the patient simply may have a prominent gland. This is sometimes recognized as a bulge below the mandibular border preoperatively but in many cases is masked by overlying fat and platysma (**Fig. 2**). Once the neck has been reshaped by liposuction or submentoplasty, the gland may be much more noticeable and a concern for the patient. Preoperative recognition and counseling of the possibility of this is important. After liposuction, the gland may present as a firm noticeable mass in the neck and can occur unilaterally or bilaterally. Treatment of this problem can be difficult. Some surgeons have tried suture resuspension techniques at the time of face-lift surgery with limited success. Another option is partial resection of the superficial portion of the submandibular gland.

Superficial resection of the gland can be performed through a submental skin incision approximately 3 cm in length. The technique is difficult and not recommended unless the surgeon already is very adept at doing a submentoplasty procedure. After making the incision a large skin flap is raised and the platysma is exposed. Subplatysmal flaps are elevated using electrocautery and the gland is usually easily noticeable if it is bulging or ptotic. Blunt dissection with a hemostat helps expose the submandibular gland. It is then grasped with a long forceps and the superficial portion can then be amputated slowly with electrocautery. Caution must be taken to avoid deep transection of the gland while working through a distant and small anterior incision, because bleeding from even a small branch of the facial artery or vein can be difficult to deal with from this limited access. Injury to the marginal mandibular branch is always a concern but unless the surgeon is overly aggressive permanent nerve injury is not common. Closure of the cervical fascia perforation over the residual gland with 2–0 Vicryl can be performed with a single interrupted suture. The closure of fascia over the gland is not absolutely necessary but may decrease the chance of postoperative hematoma, sialoceles, or recurrent gland ptosis. Once again, this procedure is for experienced surgeons and has a definite learning curve.

SIALOCELE

Sialoceles, although relatively uncommon (<0.5%), are certainly more frequent after a partial submandibular gland resection with a submentoplasty. Treatment may involve serial needle aspiration and pressure dressings. If there is doubt in distinguishing the fluid from a seroma, the fluid can be sent to test for the presence of amylase. Medical treatment for a sialocele includes the use of an anti-sialogogue or the injection of botulinum toxin A into the submandibular gland.[18,19] Sialoceles very rarely require surgical management unless the volume does not continue to decrease or if the overlying skin integrity is compromised.

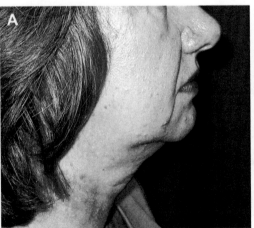
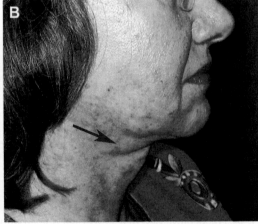

Fig. 2. (*A*) Preoperative view of a 55-year-old woman who did not want a facelift but instead underwent isolated neck liposuction. (*B*) The postoperative picture shows the untreated submandibular gland ptosis (*arrow*).

NERVE INJURY

Liposuction of the jowls and neck can result in transient weakness of the marginal mandibular branch of the facial nerve. Permanent injury is unlikely with microcannular liposuction unless the operator is overzealous or uses a cannula tip design that could potentially cut the nerve. Injury to the marginal mandibular nerve is much more common with a submentoplasty compared with liposuction. The nerve is at greatest risk if subplatysmal flaps are elevated to access the submandibular gland. In my experience, marginal mandibular nerve injury occurs less than 1% of the time. Fortunately, all of these resolved without any intervention. The incidence of facial nerve injury in face-lift surgery is reported from 0.5% to 1.7%.[20] As long as the surgeon does not suspect transection of the nerve, the only thing to do is wait for resolution. In the event of unilateral neuropraxia, the surgeon can inject 15 units of botulinum toxin to the depressors of the lip on the unaffected side to provide symmetry. It is wise to wait 4 to 6 weeks before doing this because function may return when swelling subsides.

SKIN SLOUGH

Traditional microcannular liposuction of the neck and jowls is unlikely to result in skin loss; however, use of ultrasonic or laser-assisted liposuction can create this problem (**Fig. 3**). The purported advantage of ultrasonic or laser liposuction is that the heating of the underside of the dermis results in increased collagen formation and better skin retraction following liposuction. Ultrasonic liposuction is well suited for larger areas on the body where disruption of the fat cells by cavitation can increase the efficiency of fat removal. In the neck the fat is not as abundant and it is much easier to overheat the port site or the areas being liposuctioned resulting in a thermal burn. In body liposuction, skin necrosis from internal ultrasonic liposuction has been reported to be as high as 10%.[21]

Laser liposuction using yttrium-aluminum-garnet laser technology has recently become popular. The lasers are marketed as providing better skin retraction with less bleeding or bruising and shorter recovery times. For small deposits of fat the laser-assisted liposuction techniques can be helpful. The expense of the equipment limits the

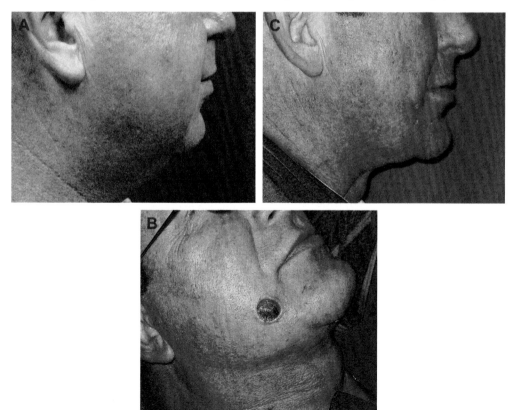

Fig. 3. (A) Preoperative view of a 55-year-old man desiring an isolated neck procedure. (B) The patient underwent submentoplasty with laser-assisted liposuction of the jowls and subsequently sustained full-thickness necrosis from overzealous laser liposuction of the jowls. (C) The postoperative picture shows the result after delayed primary closure of the wound.

use to those who perform a significant amount of liposuction in their practices. As is true of all lasers, there is a learning curve and higher power settings can create burns. The injuries can range from moderate erythema and pigment changes in the skin to full-thickness necrosis. Management is the same for any burn, including local wound care, skin grafting, or delayed primary closure.

BLEEDING AND HEMATOMAS

Using a tumescent technique, the likelihood of hematomas after facial liposuction is rare. In the event that a hematoma occurs early after surgery, the area can be anesthetized and a liposuction microcannula can be inserted to evacuate it. Compression dressings and ice may help prevent recurrence. Use of external ultrasound may help with discomfort and speed the resolution of induration.

The most common area to encounter bleeding during submentoplasty is from the anterior jugular veins in the midline of the neck and can be simply managed by suture ligation. If partial submandibular resection is performed it is possible to encounter the facial artery and vein. Controlling hemorrhage from the facial vessels from the submandibular incision can be extremely difficult. If uncontrolled bleeding in this area occurs, the surgeon may need to access the area directly over the bleeding in the submandibular region.

Small hematoma in face-lift surgery is reported to occur at an incidence of less than 15%.[22] The hallmark for expanding hematomas requiring surgical drainage is pain uncontrolled by pain medication. Large hematomas in submentoplasty are not common but could occur. My practice has a hematoma incidence for submentoplasty less than 3%. Surgical evacuation of any large hematomas and placement of a drain is the usual treatment. Small hematomas can sometimes be aspirated by a large-bore needle under local anesthesia in the office. In my experience, the use of tumescent anesthesia seems to minimize the incidence of hematomas in submentoplasty, although the literature seems to indicate that there is no lower rate of hematoma formation by using it.[6] Drains are not typically used in submentoplasty and a light compression dressing is used for 24 hours. After that, the patient wears an elastic head wrap for 2 weeks.

SEROMA

Raising a large skin flap or extensive undermining from liposuction can also result in the formation of a seroma. Blood plasma accumulation in the dead space requires aspiration or the patient can develop altered skin retraction and fibrosis in the area. Seromas are reported to occur at a rate of less than 3% with facial liposuction.[22] Serial needle aspiration and compression dressings generally take care of the problem.

POSTINFLAMMATORY HYPERPIGMENTATION

Patients with Fitzpatrick skin type III or greater are more prone to development of hyperpigmentation after liposuction. The hyperpigmentation usually resolves without any intervention, but it may take 6 months or more. The patient may apply hydroquinone 4% or kojic acid creams to the affected areas to help speed the resolution.

INFECTION

Infection is a rare occurrence in both liposuction and submentoplasty. Appropriate perioperative antibiotics and good surgical technique prevent most infections. Standard culture and sensitivities determine antibiotic therapy if infection arises. The most common organisms are streptococcus and staphylococcus introduced from the skin flora. The surgeon should also consider the possibility of methicillin-resistant *Staphylococcus aureus* because more and more cases are being reported. Community-acquired methicillin-resistant *S aureus* tends to be sensitive to fluoroquinolones and trimethoprim-sulfamethoxazole; however, health care associated methicillin-resistant *S aureus* tends to have multidrug resistance and culture and sensitivities direct antibiotic therapy.

Necrotizing fasciitis is extremely rare bacterial infection but is possible following any surgical procedure. The most common form involves group A β-hemolytic streptococci, although polymicrobial forms are possible. The hallmarks of this are significant pain uncontrolled by medication and rapidly progressive erythema, bronzing of skin, and bullae formation. Treatment involves aggressive surgical debridement, hospitalization, and intravenous antibiotics. Hyperbaric oxygen and intravenous Ig therapy are considered experimental treatment at this time.[23]

SCARRING

Scarring and poor skin retraction is most commonly an unfortunate consequence of poor patient selection or poor surgical technique. If the surgeon does not leave a sufficient amount of fat evenly distributed on the skin flaps in submentoplasty the skin may not redrape smoothly. If a hematoma or seroma forms and is not treated, significant fibrosis resulting in irregularities can occur.

SKIN REDUNDANCY

Skin redundancy is usually the result of performing liposuction or a submentoplasty on a patient with poor skin elasticity. Typically, male patients are unwilling to undergo traditional face-lifts and are looking for less invasive ways to improve their neck contour. In some cases, these patients are willing to accept some skin redundancy from a less invasive approach. Generally, if there is skin excess, it tends to bunch in the midline (**Fig. 4**). The treatments include performing a formal face-lift or direct excision with a z-plasty (**Fig. 5**).[24] Once again, some men would rather have a scar under the chin and on the neck than have the incisions of a face-lift. It is important to use a z-plasty technique to avoid linear contracture and scar band formation.

CHRONIC PAIN

Chronic pain is generally not seen with facial liposuction but can occur after submentoplasty in rare cases. After platysmaplasty the patient may report tightness in the neck and pain on swallowing. This is usually from suturing the muscle down to the hyoid fascia. This usually resolves within a couple of months. The use of medications, such as neurontin, Elavil, and Lyrica, may be helpful for the management of chronic pain.[25] In severe cases the surgeon may need to release the corset suture.

PREVENTION OF COMPLICATIONS WITH CERVICOFACIAL LIPOSUCTION

The patient should be marked before surgery with a permanent marker in an upright position to note

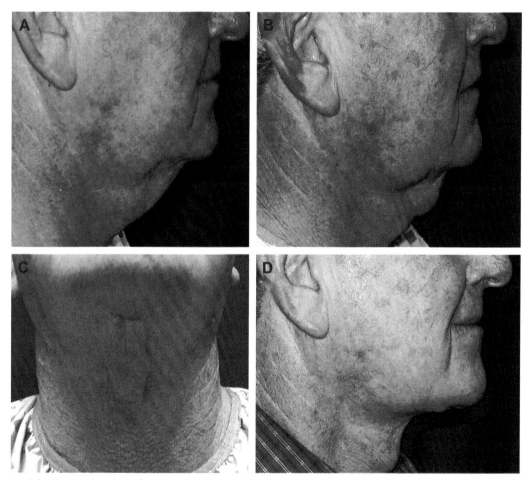

Fig. 4. (*A*) Preoperative view of a 65-year-old man with poor skin tone and skin laxity who declined having a face-lift and elected for submentoplasty alone. (*B*) Postoperatively the patient developed skin bunching in the midline of the neck. (*C*) Submental view of the skin bunching in the midline before z-plasty. (*D*) The patient elected to have a z-plasty in the midline of the neck rather than a traditional facelift. The final picture depicts the postoperative result after a z-plasty.

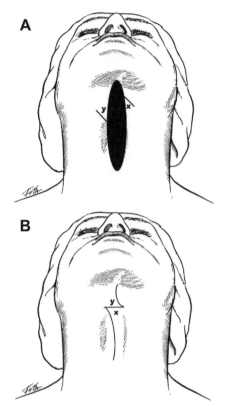

Fig. 5. (*A*) The black ellipse and lines depicts the skin excision and incisions for a z-plasty for correction of midline skin excess in patients who do not wish to have traditional facelift surgery and are willing to accept a midline neck scar. (*B*) Diagram showing the skin closure of the z-plasty. The z-plasty can be performed on both the platysma and skin but should be done in two separate layers. In cases of poorly defined platysma, the muscle may be excised.

the areas requiring the greatest amount of liposuction. Once tumescent anesthesia is infiltrated it can be difficult to note the areas of greatest fullness.

After complete skin preparation, the lower face and submental region are infiltrated with tumescent anesthesia using a 22-gauge spinal needle connected to a Wells Johnson Klein pump. I typically mix 30 mL of 2% lidocaine (600 mg) with 1.5 mL of 1:1000 epinephrine (1.5 mg) into 500 mL of normal saline. This then makes a 0.12% lidocaine with 1:333,333 epinephrine. Approximately 150 to 200 mL of the solution should be injected in the lower face and neck just superficial to the SMAS and the platysma. Injection at deeper levels may injure nerves or vascular structures. If the injection is done too superficially, a peau d'orange appearance of the skin may be noted. This appearance should be avoided. There are reports of skin slough in face-lifting that is attributed to

superficial injection of tumescent solution in areas of skin undermining. Approximately 150 mL of tumescent solution is used in the submental region.

The skin is then reprepared and the patient is draped for the procedure. It is best to wait approximately 15 to 20 minutes after injecting the solution before beginning liposuction. Stab incisions are first made with a #11 scalpel blade in the submental region, and just posterior to the pinna of the ear bilaterally.

A small 2-mm microcannula should be moved in a smooth in and out motion and each time the cannula is pushed in it should enter a new location. If the cannula is kept in the same area for multiple passes, irregularities develop that can be difficult to correct. The dominant hand holds the cannula and the nondominant hand should always be held gently over the skin to feel the depth of the cannula tip. The holes for the cannula should not be directed toward the dermis because this can disturb the subdermal plexus and result in scarring and irregularities. Additionally, the surgeon should frequently stop to feel the skin to ensure even removal of fat. In the neck, the cannula tip should not be directed below the platysma. If removal of subplatysmal fat is indicated, it should be done surgically because excessive bleeding and nerve injury can result if this is performed blindly.

When performing submental liposuction it is important not to bring the liposuction cannula above the inferior border of the mandible from the submental incision. Doing this can place the facial nerve at risk. It is better to access the jowls with the liposuction cannula from the incisions below the pinna of the ear. It is important to understand that jowling is primarily a problem with descent of tissues with age and not an area of lipohypertrophy. Conservative liposuction in the area of the jowls can be beneficial but to address the problem properly the patient should have a lower face-lift. Overly aggressive liposuction of the jowl region can result in irregularities and facial nerve weakness.

PREVENTION OF COMPLICATIONS WITH SUBMENTOPLASTY

There have been many techniques described to manage the neck in a submentoplasty.[15,26–33] The techniques to be described are how the author typically performs this operation. The technique is varied based on the patient's anatomy. If there is at least fair skin tone and no platysmal banding, this patient may benefit from liposuction alone. If there is any platysmal banding, then platysmaplasty is needed.

First, tumescent anesthesia is used to insufflate approximately 150 mL for an average-size neck. The typical mixture used is 500 mL of normal saline, 30 mL of lidocaine 2%, and 1.5 mg of epinephrine. A 2- to 3-cm submental incision is then made in the natural submental crease. If the patient has a low hyoid position and a chin implant is planned, then the incision is made posterior to the submental crease. This way the incision does not become visible, because the chin implant results in the incision appearing more anterior. The dissection is carried down to the level of the platysma with a needle tip point cautery.

It is not recommended to perform liposuction first when doing a platysmaplasty because it is essential to maintain an even thickness of superficial fat attached to the dermis. When the skin is redraped there is less chance of an uneven appearance and skin rippling. Face-lift scissors are used to undermine the skin, leaving an even layer of subdermal fat. The dissection is carried inferiorly as far as the lower border of the thyroid cartilage and laterally to the posterior border of the mandible.[34] Wide skin undermining is necessary to allow proper skin redraping after treatment of the deep tissues has been addressed. Inadequate skin undermining leads to bunching after midline plication of the platysma.

A flat spatulated cannula can then be used to perform liposuction on the fat overlying the platysma under direct vision. A lighted Aufricht retractor improves visualization through the small submental incision. Any excess submental fat is then resected. A Kelly clamp or large hemostat is placed in the midline to hold the platysma and fat while a needle tip cautery or scissors is used to resect it. It is at this point when the anterior jugular veins may be encountered. Proper hemostasis must be achieved, otherwise it is very difficult to complete the operation properly and there is a greater chance of postoperative hematoma.

After resecting the midline fat, the anterior borders of the platysma and the hyoid bone are identified. The platysma is then backcut beginning at the level of the hyoid bone. The backcut is carried back an average of 5 to 7 cm with the cut staying parallel with the inferior border of the mandible and well below the inferior extent of the submandibular gland. When making this incision through platysma care should be taken not to injure the facial vessels or nerve. The platysma is undermined superior to the area backcut. If submandibular gland ptosis or gland enlargement is recognized, I often manage this by resecting the superficial portion of the gland with the needle point cautery. This procedure is difficult to do and is not recommended to the novice. Bleeding can be encountered,

which is difficult to control from such a small incision with poor access.

After mobilizing the platysma bilaterally, a corset platysmaplasty is then performed. To do this, I use a running 2–0 vicryl suture. The inferior platysma edges are plicated at the midline to the fascia over the hyoid bone. If a chin implant is to be used to camouflage a poor cervicomental angle related to low hyoid position, it is placed at this time. Dissection is carried to the periosteum of the mandible in the midline. A subperiosteal pocket is then created at the lower border of the mandible. A solid silicone implant is then placed into this pocket. It is secured to the periosteum of the inferior border of the mandible with a single 4–0 vicryl suture. After ensuring strict hemostasis, the skin is then closed with 4–0 monocryl deep and 5–0 plain gut suture on the skin.

A dressing is then placed using Reston foam 1563L (3M Medical-Surgical, St. Paul, Minnesota) and a Coban (3M Medical-Surgical, St. Paul, Minnesota) head wrap. This is worn for 24 hours. When the patient returns the next day postoperative, the wrap is removed and the patient then wears a compression garment, such as a face-lift bra. This is to be worn as much as possible, day and night during the first week. After 1 week, the patient is to wear the garment at night only for 2 more weeks.

SUMMARY

Poor neck contour is a frequent complaint of patients. Often the most appropriate procedure is a cervicofacial rhytidectomy; however, there are instances where a less aggressive and perhaps minimally invasive procedure can provide good esthetic results. The patient with isolated submental fat deposits with good skin tone and minimal platysmal laxity may benefit from liposuction alone. Even patients who refuse a face-lift and have significant platysmal banding and laxity can have dramatic improvement with submentoplasty alone. Naturally, patients must be informed that they may require additional procedures if these isolated techniques are not completely effective to treat their problem. Limitations aside, isolated neck liposuction with or without associated submentoplasty can be a superb minimally invasive cosmetic procedure. The appropriate patient appreciates the improved neck appearance coupled with a decreased downtime as compared with traditional neck or face-lift techniques.

REFERENCES

1. Singer DP, PK S. Submandibular gland I: an anatomic evaluation and surgical approach to

submandibular gland resection for facial rejuvenation. Plast Reconstr Surg 2003;112:1150–4.

2. Gryskiewicz JM. Submental suction-assisted lipectomy without platysmaplasty: pushing the (skin) envelope to avoid a face lift for unsuitable candidates. Plast Reconstr Surg 2003;112:1406–7.

3. Hanke CW, Bullock S, Bernstein G. Current status of tumescent liposuction in the United States. National survey results. Dermatol Surg 1996;22:595–8.

4. Hanke CW, Coleman III WP. Morbidity and mortality related to liposuction: questions and answers. Dermatol Clin 1999;17:899–902.

5. Housman TS, Lawrence N, Mellen BG, et al. The safety of liposuction: results of a national survey. Dermatol Surg 2002;28:971–8.

6. Jones BM, Grover R. Reducing complications in cervicofacial rhytidectomy by tumescent infiltration: a comparative trial evaluating 678 consecutive face lifts. Plast Reconstr Surg 2004;113:398–403.

7. LaTrenta GS TM. Tumescent cervicofacial rhytidectomy. Perspectives in Plastic Surgery 2001;15:47–60.

8. Adamson PA, Cormier R, Tropper GJ, et al. Cervicofacial liposuction: results and controversies. J Otolaryngol 1990;19:267–73.

9. Bank DE, MI P. Skin retraction after liposuction in patients over the age of 40. Dermatol Surg 1999;25:673–6.

10. Chrisman BB. Liposuction with facelift surgery. Dermatol Clin 1990;8:501–22.

11. Daher JC, Cosac OM, SD. Face-lift: the importance of redefining facial contours through facial liposuction. Ann Plast Surg 1988;21:1–10.

12. Dedo DD. Liposuction of the head and neck. Otolaryngol Head Neck Surg 1987;97:591–2.

13. Goodstein WA. Superficial liposculpture of the face and neck. Plast Reconstr Surg 1996;98:988–96.

14. Grotting JC, Beckenstein MS. Cervicofacial rejuvenation using ultrasound-assisted lipectomy. Plast Reconstr Surg 2001;107:847–55.

15. Jacob CI, Berkes BJ, Kaminer MS. Liposuction and surgical recontouring of the neck: a retrospective of the neck: a retrospective analysis. Dermatol Surg 2000;26:625–32.

16. O'Ryan F, Schendel S, Poor D. Submental-submandibular suction lipectomy: indications and surgical technique. Oral Surg Oral Med Pathol 1989;67:117–25.

17. Rohrich RJ, Rios JL, Smith PD, et al. Neck rejuvenation revisited. Plast Reconstr Surg 2006;118:1251–63.

18. Capaccio P, Cuccarini V, Benicchio V, et al. Treatment of iatrogenic submandibular sialocele with botulinum toxin. Case report. Br J Oral Maxillofac Surg 2007;45:415–7.

19. Lim M, Mace A, Nouraei SA, et al. Botulinum toxin in the management of sialorrhoea: a systematic review. Clin Otolaryngol 2006;31:267–72.

20. Daane SP, Owsley JQ. Incidence of cervical branch injury with marginal mandibular nerve pseudo-paralysis in patients undergoing face lift. Plast Reconstr Surg 2003;111:2414–8.

21. Omranifard M. Ultrasonic liposuction versus surgical lipectomy. Aesthetic Plast Surg 2003;27:143–5.

22. Sullivan CA, Masin J, Maniglia AJ, et al. Complications of rhytidectomy in an otolaryngology training program. Laryngoscope 1999;109:198–203.

23. Carter PS, Banwell PE. Necrotising fasciitis: a new management algorithm based on clinical classification. Int Wound J 2004;1:189–98.

24. Zins JE, Fardo D. The anterior-only approach to neck rejuvenation: an alternative to face lift surgery. Plast Reconstr Surg 2005;115:1761–8.

25. Jensen TS, Finnerup NB. Management of neuropathic pain. Curr Opin Support Palliat Care 2007;1:126–31.

26. Feldman JJ. Corset platysmaplasty. Clin Plast Surg 1992;19:369–82.

27. Giampapa VC, Di Bernardo BE. Neck recontouring with suture suspension and liposuction: an alternative for the early rhytidectomy candidate. Aesthetic Plast Surg 1995;19:217–23.

28. Jasin ME. Submentoplasty as an isolated rejuvenative procedure for the neck. Arch Facial Plast Surg 2003;5:180–3.

29. Kamer FM. Isolated platysmaplasty: a useful procedure but with important limitations. Arch Facial Plast Surg 2003;5:184.

30. Kamer FM, Frankel AS. Isolated submentoplasty: a limited approach to the aging neck. Arch Otolaryngol Head Neck Surg 1997;123:66–70.

31. Kamer FM, Lefkott LA. Submental surgery: a graduated approach to the aging neck. Arch Otolaryngol Head Neck Surg 1991;117:40–6.

32. Knize DM. Limited incision submental lipectomy and platysmaplasty. Plast Reconstr Surg 1998;101:473–81.

33. Knize DM. Limited incision submental lipectomy and platysmaplasty. Plast Reconstr Surg 2004;113:1275–8.

34. Ramirez OM. Cervicoplasty: nonexcisional anterior approach. Plast Reconstr Surg 1997;99:1576–85.

Complications Following Fat Transfer

Robert A. Glasgold, MD[a,b,*], Mark J. Glasgold, MD, FACS[a,b],
Samuel M. Lam, MD, FACS[c]

KEYWORDS

• Fat grafting • Complications • Fat transfer

Traditionally, strategies for facial rejuvenation have emphasized correction of tissue ptosis and laxity with suspensory and excisional techniques, such as face-lifting and blepharoplasty. Volume loss plays a significant role in facial aging and, until recently, had not received appropriate attention. Facial fat grafting to correct volume loss has become a crucial component of facial rejuvenation in the authors' respective practices.[1]

Fat grafting has had a long and controversial history, owing principally to failed past techniques that have left a trail of problems in their wake. Fat grafting complications are generally related to either contour abnormalities or issues of longevity/predictability. Most contour problems can be avoided using appropriate injection techniques. This article reviews a stepwise approach to dealing with contour irregularities. Variability of results, in terms of longevity and predictability, are inherent with the use of fat grafting (**Fig. 1**A, B). During the preoperative consultation, realistic expectations must be established, emphasizing the variability in results and the possible need for multiple procedures to achieve the desired outcome (**Fig. 2**A–C).

COMPLICATIONS INVOLVING LONGEVITY

Perhaps one of the major reasons many surgeons have been reluctant to adopt facial fat grafting as a surgical treatment option is the perceived transience of the result. Many surgeons have tried and given up on facial fat grafting because of failed attempts to achieve any durability. The authors feel that the reason for this failure, or perceived failure, stems from two problems: placing fat into facial areas that are not ideally treated with fat grafting and poor operative technique.

The two areas most commonly treated with fat grafting are the lips and facial lines, particularly the nasolabial and labiomandibular folds. These areas represent the zones with the poorest retention of fat. Poor survival of transferred adipocytes to these locations is generally attributed to the hyperdynamic nature of these recipient sites.

Although durable and beautiful results can be achieved with fat grafting into one's lips, two problems arise with this method: the poor take of adipocytes and a protracted recovery time. Patients undergoing lip augmentation using fat tend to be unhappy in the shorter term because of the prolonged distorted appearance caused by edema, and in the long term feel the result is less than they hoped for, especially factoring in their downtime. In the nasolabial and labiomandibular folds, prolonged postoperative recovery is not as significant an issue; patient dissatisfaction is generally related to the limited improvement once the swelling resolves. For these reasons, in patients whose primary goal is lip augmentation or filling of facial rhytids, the authors' preference is to use off-the-shelf injectables (ie, hyaluronic acid) rather than fat transfer.

For patients undergoing fat transfer for volume augmentation in other regions of the face, it is worthwhile to address the nasolabial and labiomandibular folds. Treating these areas does not prolong recovery time and, as long as patients

[a] Department of Surgery, University of Medicine & Dentistry of New Jersey, Robert Wood Johnson Medical School, Piscataway, NJ, USA
[b] Glasgold Group Plastic Surgery, 31 River Road, Highland Park, NJ 08904, USA
[c] Willow Bend Wellness Center, Lam Facial Plastic Surgery Center & Hair Restoration Institute, 6101 Chapel Hill Boulevard, Suite 101, Plano, TX 75093, USA
* Corresponding author.
E-mail address: drrobert@glasgoldgroup.com (R.A. Glasgold).

Oral Maxillofacial Surg Clin N Am 21 (2009) 53–58
doi:10.1016/j.coms.2008.10.004
1042-3699/08/$ – see front matter © 2009 Elsevier Inc. All rights reserved.

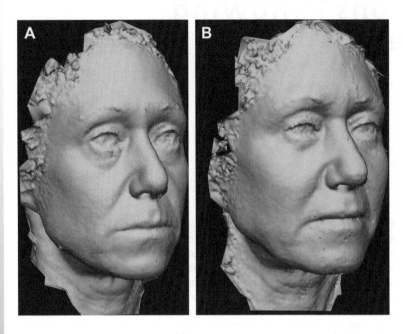

Fig. 1. Long-term result is shown in this patient using the Vectra 3D System (Canfield Scientific, Fairfield, New Jersey). Preoperative (*A*) and 2 years postoperative (*B*) contour images are shown in this patient who underwent a single midface (inferior orbital rim and cheek) fat transfer procedure. The 3D Vectra system allows for volume comparison; this patient shows persistence of result with retention of 35% of the injected volume at 2-year follow-up.

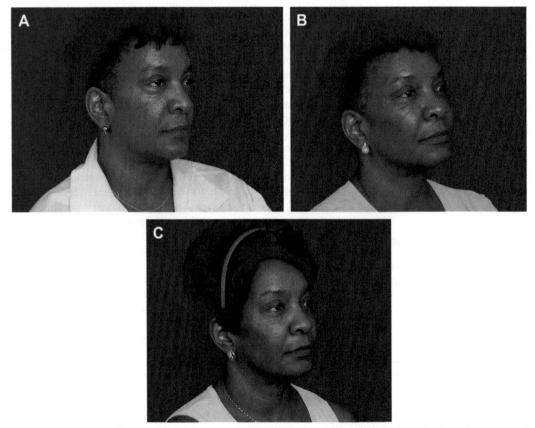

Fig. 2. Large-volume midface augmentation requiring multiple fat transfers to obtain desired result. Preoperative (*A*), 5 months after initial surgery (*B*), and 1-year after second fat transfer (*C*) showing the desired correction. (*From* Lam SM, Glasgold MJ, Glasgold RA. Complementary fat grafting. Philadelphia: Lippincott Williams & Wilkins; 2007. p. 94; with permission.)

understand the limitations, are likely to provide some improvement.

A second possible reason for poor fat retention is related to surgical technique. Numerous fat grafting techniques have proven reliable in achieving superior long-term results.[2] Several key technical points should be emphasized to optimize results of the surgery. The authors believe that atraumatic harvesting of fat, centrifugation to isolate the fat (eg, removing blood, lidocaine), and fat injection in small parcels all contribute to improved adipocyte survival. Machine liposuction in which fat is removed under high pressure is more traumatic to the adipocytes and may contribute to poorer survival of the transferred cells. The authors' preference is to harvest fat with a 10-mL Luer-Lok syringe maintaining approximately 2 to 3 cm³ of negative pressure. Before injecting fat, the fat is isolated using centrifugation (2000–3000 rpm for 1–2 minutes) (**Fig. 3**). After centrifugation, the fatty-acid supranatant is poured off and the bloody infranatant drained. The column of fat is then transferred into individual 1-mL Luer-Lok syringes for infiltration (**Fig. 4**).

Fat injections are performed using 1-mL Luer-Lok syringes outfitted with only blunt cannulas (Tulip, San Diego, California) (**Fig. 5**). The fat is injected in small parcels in many different layers to increase the surface area of injected fat exposed to vascularized tissue. Blunt cannulas reduce localized tissue trauma in the recipient sites and theoretically should improve fat take. Finally, limiting the amount of fat transferred may enhance the percentage of fat that survives. If an excessive amount of fat is injected into a single site, a greater portion of nonvascularized donor adipocytes are

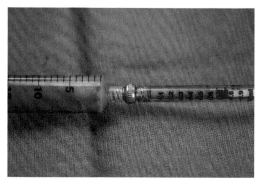

Fig. 4. Transfer of fat into 1-mL Luer-Lok syringes in preparation for fat injections. (*From* Lam SM, Glasgold MJ, Glasgold RA. Complementary fat grafting. Philadelphia: Lippincott Williams & Wilkins; 2007. p. 58; with permission.)

probably being placed adjacent to each other, potentially reducing adipocyte survival.

COMPLICATIONS INVOLVING CONTOUR PROBLEMS
Avoiding Complications

Before discussing treatment of a complication, why they occur and how to avoid them should be explored. The authors previously encountered problems in the inferior orbital rim, where most fat-related contour problems occur. The major reason for this complication was rooted in the orientation of the cannula to the orbital rim. Early in their experience they had placed fat along the inferior orbital rim, entering from the lateral canthal region, placing fat in a plane parallel to the rim. This approach led to numerous contour problems that have subsequently been avoided through layering fat across the inferior orbital rim in a perpendicular orientation (**Fig. 6**).

The infiltration cannula enters from a midcheek stab incision with the fat being deposited in

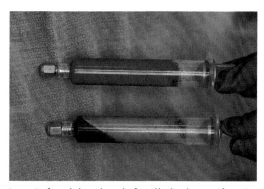

Fig. 3. Before (*above*) and after (*below*) centrifugation of harvested fat. Centrifugation isolates the fat from blood, lidocaine, and other nonviable components of the harvested material. (*From* Lam SM, Glasgold MJ, Glasgold RA. Complementary fat grafting. Philadelphia: Lippincott Williams & Wilkins; 2007. p. 56; with permission.)

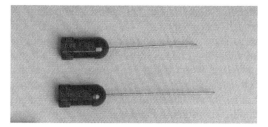

Fig. 5. Blunt fat infiltration cannulas. The 0.9 mm (4-cm length) is used for periorbital injections (*above*). The 1.2 mm (6-cm length) is used for all other regions. (*From* Lam SM, Glasgold MJ, Glasgold RA. Complementary fat grafting. Philadelphia: Lippincott Williams & Wilkins; 2007. p. 44; with permission.)

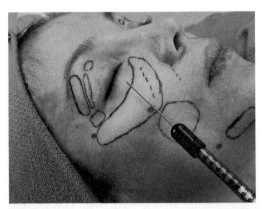

Fig. 6. Intraoperative display of approach for injecting the inferior orbital rim. The cannula entry point is delineated with the red mark in the midcheek. (*From* Lam SM, Glasgold MJ, Glasgold RA. Complementary fat grafting. Philadelphia: Lippincott Williams & Wilkins; 2007. p. 66; with permission.)

a supraperiosteal plane in tiny aliquots of 0.01 to 0.05 mL per pass. In general, 2-mL of fat are placed along the entire inferior orbital rim in a supraperiosteal plane. In patients who have more volume loss, another 1 to 2 mL of fat are placed more superficial but always remaining deep to the orbicularis oculi muscle. A more superficial and higher-volume treatment is more safely performed with greater experience injecting this area. This conservative approach will help avoid overcorrection. Given that undercorrection is much easier to address than overcorrection, the best plan is to "hit doubles" rather than trying to "score a home run." Hence, avoiding complications should be the goal of any fat transfer, especially by neophyte surgeons embarking on this new surgical venture.

Treating Complications

Many types of potential complications can arise after fat transfer, including reported incidences of infection, nerve injury, and arterial embolism. Although extremely rare cases of embolism and nerve injury have been reported, the authors believe that the chance of these occurring is further minimized when using blunt injection cannulas.[3] With meticulous sterile preparation and execution, the risk for infection can also be diminished significantly. The authors have encountered two cases of post–fat transfer infection; both were atypical mycobacteria and both resolved with appropriate antibiotics. The more likely types of fat transfer complications that may be encountered are contour problems, particularly in the periorbital region. To make treatment strategies more

straightforward, they have divided the types of contour complications into the following entities: lumps, bulges, persistent malar edema, overcorrection, undercorrection, and divoting at the cannula entry site.

Lumps

A lump is defined as a small, discrete mass of injected fat that may occur for two reasons. First, the lump may arise if too large a bolus of fat is placed in a sensitive region like the lower eyelid. Second, the fat may have been placed too superficially so that it becomes visible as a contour deformity. Although steroid injections may be a reasonable first step, these lumps may need to be excised to achieve complete resolution. If excision is required in the lower lid region, the most discreet placement for an incision is in the tear trough at the junction of the thin lower lid skin and thicker sebaceous cheek skin (**Fig. 7**A–D).

Bulges

Although at first glance a bulge may seem to be the same as a lump, the authors make a distinction to guide treatment strategy. A bulge is typified by a wider, cigar-roll appearance along the inferior orbital rim that can arise from three causes. First, the bulge could arise from imprecise placement of fat along the inferior orbital rim, usually from a lateral entry point. This type of bulge is characterized by a fibrotic and indurated nature and readily responds to injectable agents that can reduce the element of scarring, such as 5-fluoruouracil and dilute triamcinalone acetonide.

Another type of bulge can arise in the lateral aspect of the malar region and may be caused by overcorrection. This bulge is more apparent when the patient smiles. The most targeted solution to address this problem is focused microliposuction to reduce the bulk of fat in this area. Finally, a bulge may develop when the patient gains excessive weight. The best way to mitigate this problem is through weight loss.

Persistent Malar Mound Edema

Persistent swelling in the malar region should be distinguished from either a bulge or overcorrection. The malar mound is a triangular-shaped elevation, anatomically delineated by the orbital septal–periosteal adhesion superiorly and the malar septum inferiorly (**Fig. 8**).[4] The most important step in avoiding this complication is to identify the presence of a malar mound preoperatively and determine whether the patient has a history of cyclical swelling. For these patients, careful explanation of this potential problem is very important.

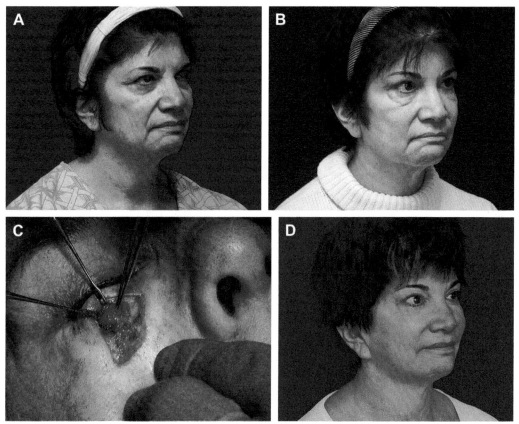

Fig. 7. (*A*) Patient before fat transfer to the inferior orbital rim and cheek. (*B*) At 6 months postoperatively, patient had a lump in the central inferior orbital rim and was also unhappy with the residual lateral fat pad. (*C*) Intraoperative photograph showing removal of the lump of transplanted fat that was causing the contour irregularity. This incision, at the junction of the lower lid and cheek skin, allowed for removal of redundant lower-lid skin. At the same setting, the lateral fat pad was reduced through a transconjunctival approach. (*D*) Postoperative photograph, after correction of the contour irregularity. (*From* Lam SM, Glasgold MJ, Glasgold RA. Complementary fat grafting. Philadelphia: Lippincott Williams & Wilkins; 2007. p. 90; with permission.)

Intraoperatively, avoiding placement of fat in the malar mound can lessen the chance of this problem. Persistent malar mound edema generally occurs only in patients who have a visibly defined malar mound preoperatively, especially if they have a history of cyclical malar mound edema. Although the condition may resolve independently over time, if it persists, dilute steroid (kenalog) injections repeated every 4 to 6 weeks as necessary may hasten this process. In rare cases, a malar mound that preoperatively exhibits abnormal overlying skin and marked edema, may be better managed with direct excision of the malar mound.

Overcorrection

Overcorrection is best avoided through a conservative fat transfer. "Hitting doubles" should underscore every fat-grafting endeavor, especially for surgeons just starting out and unsure of how much of the fat will take and how much to inject.

If the transplanted area looks overcorrected, waiting a minimum of 6 months before intervention is advisable to allow for resolution of edema or resorption of fat over time. If this fails, then microliposuction of the overcorrected area may be required.

Undercorrection

Undercorrection is definitely the easiest contour problem to correct and should be anticipated in every patient. All patients are counseled on the likely chance that a second fat transfer procedure will be needed to obtain the ideal result. Placing additional fat is a very easy task compared with the onerous one of extraction. The need for secondary fat transfer is seen more frequently in patients requiring large volume augmentation, those who smoke, and those who are extreme exercisers.

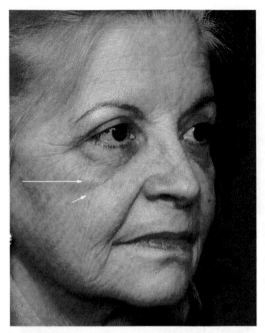

Fig. 8. The malar mound is a triangular-shaped elevation (*large arrow*), anatomically delineated by the orbital septal–periosteal adhesion superiorly and the malar septum inferiorly (*small arrow*). (*From* Lam SM, Glasgold MJ, Glasgold RA. Complementary fat grafting. Philadelphia: Lippincott Williams & Wilkins; 2007. p. 14; with permission.)

Divoting at the Injection Site

This contour problem is extremely infrequent and is characterized by skin tethering to the deeper tissues at the injection site. Subcising this adherence with a 20-gauge needle can usually manage the problem. Occasionally, fillers such as hyaluronic acids may be needed to stent this area during the healing phase to minimize relapse.

SUMMARY

Fat grafting has truly become a reliable and consistent method of long-term volume correction that is mandated to rejuvenate most aging faces. Prior techniques that led to short-lived longevity and poor outcomes have been superseded by modern methods that ensure excellent results in most patients. The hope is that understanding the pearls and pitfalls presented in this article will help prospective surgeons not only treat complications that follow fat grafting but also avoid them initially.

REFERENCES

1. Lam SM, Glasgold MJ, Glasgold RA. Complementary fat grafting. Philadelphia, PA: Lippincott, Williams, Wilkins; 2007.
2. Shiffman MA, Mirrafati S. Fat transfer techniques: the effect of harvest and transfer methods on adipocyte viability and review of the literature. Dermatol Surg 2001;27(9):819–26.
3. Coleman SR. Structural fat grafting. St. Louis, (MO): Quality Medical Publishing, Inc.; 2004.
4. Mendelson BC, Muzaffar AR, Adams WP. Surgical anatomy of the midcheek and malar mounds. Plast Reconstr Surg 2002;110(3):885–96.

Complications in Facelift Surgery and Their Prevention

Joseph Niamtu III, DMD

KEYWORDS

- Complications in facelift surgery
- Complications in Rhytidectomy
- Cosmetic facial surgery complications
- Facelift • Rhytidectomy

There is little argument that facelift surgery (rhytidectomy) is the ultimate rejuvenative procedure. Although there are many "new" facelift techniques, in reality, they have been around for almost a century and have undergone numerous refinements that are used today.[1–14] Of all cosmetic procedures, none are more life changing or visibly exposed in everyday life. A natural-appearing facelift can literally change a patient's life in innumerable ways. It can make a patient not only look younger but feel younger, which can have an impact on his or her entire affect. Contrarily, an unnatural facelift or one with significant complications can have a negative impact on the patient's appearance and attitude. It can also harm the doctor's reputation and cause lawsuits. Although no surgeon can guarantee a procedure without complications, most facelift complications are predictable and frequently avoidable by obeying sound pre-, intra-, and postoperative techniques. Even the best surgeon, with the best patient, with the best anesthesiologist and surgical team can and is likely to experience complications associated with facelift surgery.

The purpose of this article is not to be an authoritative analysis of technique with strict dogma but rather to discuss the pros and cons of various aspects of rhytidectomy surgery. Much of what is said by any surgeon can be disputed by another. What may work well in the hands of one surgeon may falter in the hands of another. There is rarely only a single means of accomplishing anything, including facelift surgery. The true purpose of this article is to present comparisons of thought and technique that have worked well (or not) in the hands of the author. It is needless to state that others can argue, dispute, and defend techniques, and that is what makes learning and teaching an endless experience. The author therefore presents his experiences that have led to performing approximately 85 facelifts a year and what has proved beneficial along the way over the past decade in his cosmetic facial practice. Agree or disagree, it is the author's hope that he can enlighten some surgeons and, at the least, stimulate thought and discussion with those who disagree. There is not right or wrong; there is only a good result or a poor result. The bottom line of all is happy patients and a prosperous practice. All surgeons have results that are great and, every once in a while, some that we are less proud of. The trick is to maximize the aforementioned and minimize the latter.

Because it is impossible to incorporate all aspect of facelift complications into the confines of this article, the author focuses on some of the more common problematic and avoidable complications.

PREOPERATIVE CONSIDERATIONS

Intraoperative or postoperative death is, of course, the most tragic complication and sometimes happens because of circumstances beyond the surgeon's control. The best offense for such a tragedy is a good defense. This begins with picking appropriate patients for the given procedure.

Cosmetic Facial Surgery, 11319 Polo Place, Midlothian, VA 23113, USA
E-mail address: niamtu@niamtu.com

Oral Maxillofacial Surg Clin N Am 21 (2009) 59–80
doi:10.1016/j.coms.2008.10.001
1042-3699/08/$ – see front matter © 2009 Elsevier Inc. All rights reserved.

Patients undergoing facelift procedures are frequently elderly and may have multisystem disease and be on multiple medications. Most patients do well with proper medical, anesthetic, and surgical management, but some patients are clearly not suitable candidates. The surgeon's enthusiasm to operate should never supersede common sense. We must remember that no one needs a facelift; it is an elective procedure and not one worth dying for.

In the author's practice, all patients undergoing facelift procedures receive a thorough preoperative history and physical examination by their physician. This includes an electrocardiogram, chest radiograph if indicated, and appropriate blood and coagulation studies. In addition, the anesthesiologist reviews the charts of any questionable patients a week before the procedure. Although most patients totally understand the necessity of a thorough workup, a patient occasionally balks at the hassle; in this case, the author convinces or dismisses that individual. The liability outweighs the procedure.

Patients who have controlled hypertension or diabetes are most often cleared and fare well. Patients with cardiac or respiratory problems prevent more of a risk. Patients with a history of previous angina or coronary artery disease must receive significant preoperative work by a cardiologist and frequently undergo cardiac CT and a stress test, for example. Important information for the surgeon to acquire includes the following questions. What is the valve function? What is the ventricular function? What is the status of the coronary artery system? Is the patient arrhythmogenic?

Patients who have emphysema must undergo pulmonary consultation and related tests, such as a pulmonary function test. Ultimately, every medically compromised patient is a calculated risk, and the more consultations performed before surgery, the better. With medically compromised patients, aggressive or multiple procedures may be better avoided in exchange for more conservative or singular procedures.

Smokers present well-known surgical and anesthetic risks. Anesthetically, they have increased secretions, more reactive airways, decreased lung capacity, and oxygenation problems. After surgery, they are more at risk for tissue necrosis and delayed healing. Some surgeons refuse to operate on smokers. The author practices in Richmond, Virginia, which is the headquarters for Philip Morris, and Virginia is a huge tobacco-growing state. Many of his patients smoke. Getting them to quit is usually futile, and even if they say they quit, the author assumes that they have not. He uses a specialized smoker's consent form, which details the various problems associated with smoking and surgery. He also performs a more conservative procedure on these patients. Whereas he may simultaneously laser normal patients undergoing facelift procedures, he may refrain from concomitant laser resurfacing so as not to stress the lipocutaneous flap in smokers. The author can honestly say that in the many smokers on whom he has performed facelift surgery, their complication rate is no greater than that of his nonsmoking population. This may be luck or coincidence, but he thinks that smoking is not an absolute contraindication to rhytidectomy.

Deep vein thrombosis (DVT; or resultant pulmonary embolus) is a problem that may occur in longer operations, such as a facelift. Combining a facelift with other cosmetic facial procedures can lead to 5- to 6-hour cases of immobilization during anesthesia. Obese patients, medically compromised patients, patients on birth control pills, and other factors can increase the incidence of DVT. The author believes that general anesthesia increases the possibility of DVT because of the absolute extended immobility of the patient. He prefers intravenous sedation because the anesthetic plane is not as deep and the patient can move his or her extremities. All the author's patients undergoing a facelift (or procedures that last longer than 2 hours) wear compression hose during surgery, and in higher risk patients or those undergoing general anesthesia, he uses pneumatic compression devices. In addition, his anesthetist and staff regularly massage and mobilize the patient's extremities to induce blood flow and prevent pressure points.

There is no substitute for ardent preoperative evaluation, testing, workup, and prevention. Something as simple as aspirin or any medication that influences platelet function can contribute to hematoma and begin a cascade of resultant complications.

INTRAOPERATIVE COMPLICATIONS

Problems that occur during the operation include surgical and anesthetic considerations. The airway is always the prime consideration with any anesthetic. There are arguments for and against an intubated airway, and this depends on multiple factors between the anesthesiologist and surgeon. As stated previously, the author prefers intravenous conscious or deep sedation. He sometimes uses laryngeal mask airways, elongated nasal pharyngeal airways (Rusch tubes), or simple nasal oxygen cannulas. The patient's anatomy, size, respiratory status, airway obstruction, and length of surgery factor into the appropriate choice. When a noninvasive airway is used, the ability to intubate must be an ever-present consideration and the appropriate medications and equipment must be at arm's reach.

Hypertensive patients can be managed with Clonidine (Boehringer, Ridgefield, Connecticut) at a dose of 0.1 to 0.2 mg immediately before surgery to lower blood pressure. Blood pressure control throughout the surgery is important, and small doses of beta-blockers, such as Labetalol (Hospira, Inc., Lake Forest, Illinois) may be given when required. Narcotics are kept to a minimum to prevent extended recovery and postoperative nausea and vomiting. Patients who undergo procedures that last longer than 4 hours may be catheterized at the beginning of surgery.

Nerve pressure points in the extremities must also be considered because of long periods of immobilization, and adequate padding on the operating table in addition to periodic mobilizing of the extremities by the anesthetist and staff is important. These are just a few of the many considerations that require thought and preparation during surgery.

Detail to hemostasis cannot be overstated to prevent postfacelift hematoma. Some surgical procedures can be closed with minor bleeding, but a doctor who returns to the office in the middle of the night to drain a major facelift hematoma may wish that he or she paid more attention to bleeding during surgery. The surgeon must continually, throughout each step of the facelift procedure, access any bleeding and control it. Bipolar forceps with radiowave surgery or electrosurgery are indispensable in rhytidectomy.

Intraoperative Surgical Complications

Preventing complications through incision design

For all the work and expertise that goes into a facelift, the incisions are the only thing that the patients can see. The final scar is the signature of the surgeon, and all attempts at producing an imperceptible scar should be exercised. The author always makes his incision markings with the patient standing before going to the operating room. Marking a patient in the supine position can produce deceptive markings because of the effect of gravity. In addition, it is important to mark the patient before any local or tumescent anesthesia is administered because it distorts the anatomic boundaries. The lipocutaneous flap should always be treated with ultimate care and never closed under tension. The author believes that a retrotragal incision is the most cosmetic incision for women and shys away from pretragal incisions in women. Although the pretragal incision oftentimes heals with an acceptable scar, the skin color and texture differences between the cheek skin and the ear skin usually make this type of incision noticeable. Having said that, it takes significant skill to produce a natural postoperative tragus, and if the surgeon cannot perform this with regularity and precision, the pretragal approach is preferable. In male patients, especially those with a natural preauricular crease, the pretragal incision is more acceptable. It usually blends well, especially with bearded skin, and also prevents pulling bearded skin on the tragus. Again, in skilled hands, the retrotragal incision is also good in men. **Fig. 1** shows an example of both anterior incision designs.

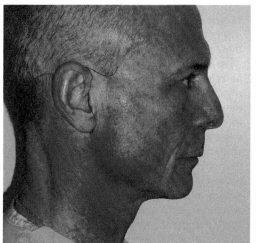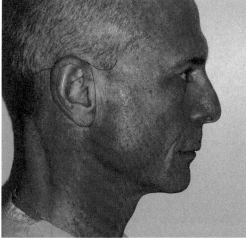

Fig. 1. Image on the left shows the retrotragal incision design that is used in women, whereas the image on the right shows the preauricular incision used only in men by the author.

Because the incision curves around the earlobe, it should be made in the natural crease at the attachment. Although some surgeons prefer to extend the incision slightly outside the natural lobe crease, the skin color and texture can be obvious. For this reason, the author prefers to place the lobe incision at its natural junction. As stated, marking the patient in the standing position before surgery provides an accurate template to incise. Attention to the postauricular incision is also important even though it is hidden. In women, some surgeons prefer to place the postauricular incision 4 to 5 mm superior to the posterior auricular sulcus with the intention of the scar contracting into the sulcus after surgery, and thus being hidden. Others contest this and simply place the incision in the depth of the sulcus. In men, placing the incision on the posterior auricular surface can be problematic because it can place bearded skin onto the back of the ear, which is problematic to shave. **Fig. 2** illustrates the incision choices for the posterior auricular incision.

Avoiding a noticeable scar behind the ear is accomplished by placing the scalp incision at its greatest point of camouflage. This corresponds to the area where the posterior hairline is closest to the helical rim, which is usually at the greatest width of the pinna. Although this involves somewhat more dissection, the scar is much less noticeable than when placed over the mastoid region (**Fig. 3**).

At the transition to the hair-bearing scalp, most surgeons extend the incision well into the hairline (at the greatest width of the pinna) with a gentle tapering or use an occipital hairline incision. Using the higher hairline incision is the author's preferred technique, but this needs careful execution so as to avoid a stepped hairline. The incision tapers off into the posterior scalp, and when pulling the skin flap into a positive vector, care needs to be taken to rotate the flap slightly anteriorly to align the natural curve of the posterior hairline (**Fig. 4**). Failure to do this can lead to the telltale step of the posterior hairline (**Fig. 5**).

Consideration also needs to be given to deciding whether to use a higher scalp incision or one that follows the natural occipital hairline. Using the latter is definitely easier and faster because it requires less scalp dissection. When this incision heals naturally, it is usually quite esthetic, but when there is dehiscence, hypertrophic scarring, or hypopigmentation (all of which can occur in the best of hands and talent), this incision is extremely noticeable and precludes the patient from wearing his or her hair up. For this reason, the author prefers the higher placed postauricular incision. Although the more superiorly placed incision is usually more esthetic, it can be problematic in patients with abundantly excessive neck skin. With significant anterior neck excess, the higher placed incision can produce posterior auricular balding because of the fact that the skin is pulled so far superiorly and the posterior hairline is significantly elevated. In patients with obviously excessive neck skin, the author prefers the lower occipital hairline incision (**Fig. 6**).

Temporal tuft incision management

As important as posterior auricular and hairline esthetics are, they can frequently be hidden, whereas the preauricular hairline is much more difficult to conceal. One of the most telltale stigmas of poor incision design is an unnatural-appearing temporal tuft and sideburn. Unfortunately, the author sees this result on a regular basis from some extremely capable local surgeons (**Fig. 7**). As stated in the introduction, the author fully realizes that one can dispute, argue, and defend a given technique, but he has consistently witnessed unnatural temporal tuft esthetics from other surgeons who use a vertical temporal incision in the preauricular temporal region. Some surgeons say that they can adjust the vector of pull so as not to produce temporal tuft elevation, but there are obviously many others who cannot. Having said

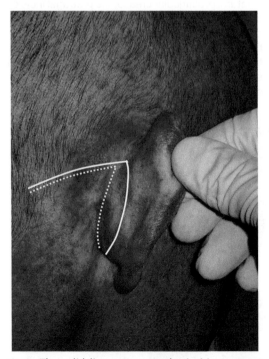

Fig. 2. The solid line represents the incision pattern used in women, whereas the dotted line is the preferred position in men.

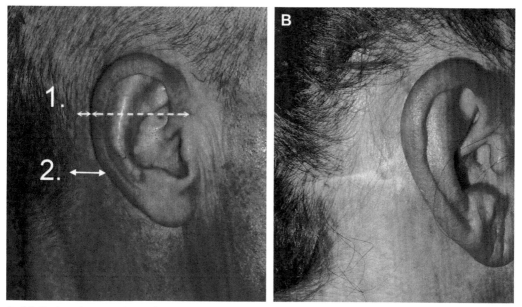

Fig. 3. (*A*) Placing the posterior scalp incision at the greatest width of the pinna makes a smaller visible scar when compared with a lower mastoid incision. (*B*) Unsightly lower mastoid scar that could have been easily camouflaged by making it in a more superior position, where the pinna meets the hairline.

this, the author designs his incision to lie just inside the natural curvature of the temporal tuft or sideburn region. There is an area of follicular density change from fine hair to a more dense "real" hairline several millimeters into the tuft, and that is where he places the incision (**Fig. 8**). Beveling this incision and cutting across the more inferior

hair follicles allow follicular regrowth into the care for concealment.

Some surgeons continue this temporal hairline incision all the way around the anterior hairline to the level of the brow, but if this scar pulls apart or otherwise heals ungracefully, it is quite noticeable. One reason to carry this incision to that

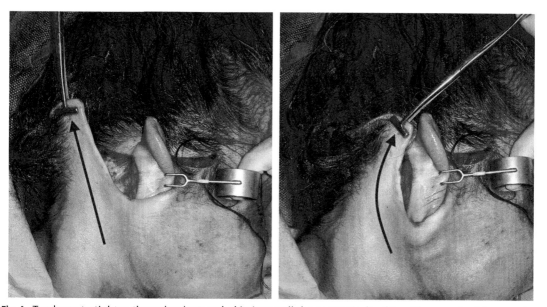

Fig. 4. Tendency to tighten the redundant neck skin is to pull the postauricular skin with a purely oblique vector. Although this dramatically tightens the neck and submental region, it can produce a step in the natural hairline curvature (*left*). The other image (*right*) shows the proper vector with a slight anterior rotation to approximate the posterior hairline more naturally.

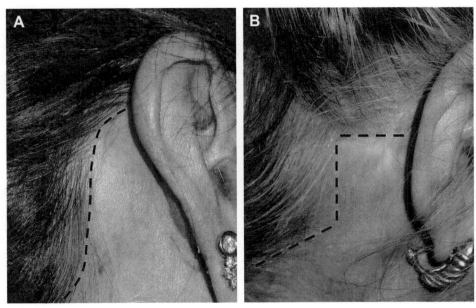

Fig. 5. (*A*) Posterior hairline with a stepped hairline attributable to failure of proper flap rotation. (*B*) Hairline with a natural arc.

degree is to be able to provide a vector of pull on the midface and even the lateral brow. A compromise in this design is instead of following the temporal tuft to its extent, to make the incision approximately 2 cm into the tuft and then to provide a vertical release within the tuft (see **Fig. 8**). The vertical release allows dissection to the canthus and also permits the surgeon to bunch the skin well into the temple (**Fig. 9**). This prevents the frequent lateral canthal bunching that can occur with a total temporal curving incision. The bunched hair in the high temple can then be adjusted with a Burrow's triangle or other method that camouflages the scar in the high hairline. With careful attention to vector direction, the natural tuft esthetics are maintained.

Addressing the superficial muscular aponeurotic system (SMAS) can be an article in itself.[15–20] The author prefers the lateral SMASectomy technique as described by Baker,[20] with certain personal modifications. He believes that this technique provides the greatest control of the deeper tissues and also provides the most secure longevity. Although some surgeons advocate aggressive sub-SMAS dissection, the author has not found this to be significantly beneficial to results. In addition to lengthening recovery, it can invite more damage to motor nerves. When dealing with the lateral SMASectomy, the author prefers to stay over the parotid gland, where the motor nerves are best protected. As the anterior border of the parotid is approached, the scissor tips are always pointed upward to avoid nerve injury. During the SMAS

excision, the mobile SMAS is "tented" by elevating with forceps to lift it from the underlying parotido-masseteric fascia (**Fig. 10**). As the facial nerve branches emerge under this facial layer, it should be the inferior limit of dissection to protect the nerve branches. The motor branches are especially

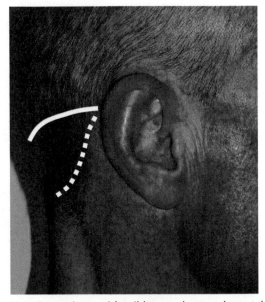

Fig. 6. For patients with mild to moderate submental skin excess, the higher placed posterior scalp incision is preferred, but when treating patients with excessive neck skin, placing the incision at the natural hairline can prevent unsightly raising of the posterior hairline.

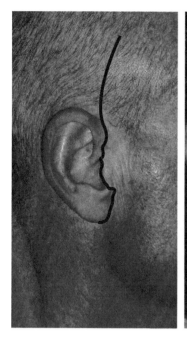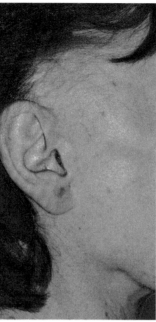

Fig. 7. An elevated temporal hairline with resulting baldness of this area is an unforgivable iatrogenic deformity and extremely problematic for patients (*right*). This type of deformity is more frequent when using a pure vertical temporal incision (*left*).

vulnerable as they cross the masseter muscle, and this technique is not recommended for the novice facelift surgeon. A rectangle of SMAS is excised in a vector parallel to the nasolabial fold, which allows the pull of the SMAS to be perpendicular to the nasolabial fold, thereby improving it (**Fig. 11**).

After excision of the SMAS rectangle, the distal and proximal SMASectomy borders are sutured as shown in **Fig. 12** (left image). The excised SMAS is overlaid on the skin to show the approximate position of the excision in **Fig. 12** (right image).

Related to this discussion of deeper dissection is the protection of the greater auricular nerve (GAN) and external jugular vein during lateral neck dissection (**Fig. 13**). The GAN crosses the

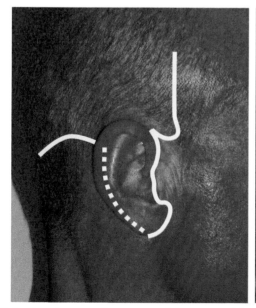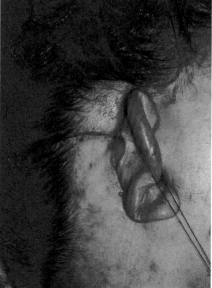

Fig. 8. Following the natural curvature of the temporal hairline can prevent unnatural elevation of this area.

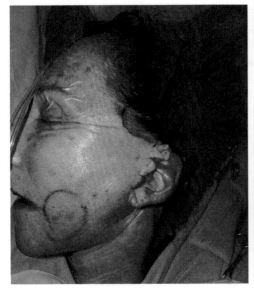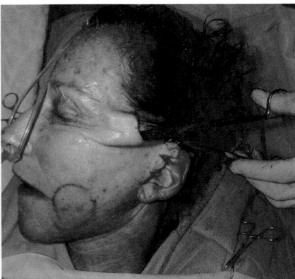

Fig. 9. Incorporating a vertical release within the temporal tuft allows positional maintenance with the ability to control lateral canthal bunching.

belly of the sternocleidomastoid muscle (SCM) approximately 6.5 cm inferior to the external auditory meatus. There is little subcutaneous fat in this region, and it is not uncommon for the SCM fascia to be intimate with the dermis in this region. For this reason, judicious dissection must be performed so as not to injure the GAN that runs superficial in this area. Adequate tumescent anesthesia assists in "ballooning" this tissue plane, as does subcutaneous "pretunneling" with a small, blunt, spatulate dissecting instrument. Dissecting with the scissor tips upward is also protective, and the surgeons and staff should always make an attempt to concentrate in this area.

Hemostasis is a prime consideration of facelift surgery, and careful attention to bleeding must be executed throughout the entire procedure. Nothing is more stressful than dealing with a postoperative expanding hematoma in the middle of the night. This is something that must be planned in advanced and anticipated for each case. Most novice surgeons have found themselves in the precarious position of having to take a patient back to the office surgery center after hours, with the stress of not being to reach their staff, the surgical instruments still being dirty in the sink, the anesthetic medications being locked up, and being alone with an anxious patient and family. An ounce of prevention is definitely worth many pounds of cure in this situation. The key is to anticipate the complication. This involves having staff on call to respond, having sterile instruments available, and having access to anesthetic medications and personnel. Having a proactive plan for dealing with

hematoma or other emergent complications is a significant necessity.

Prevention of postoperative hemorrhage is the best plan. It is difficult to attempt to "catch up" with bleeding at the end of a case, before wound closure. The astute surgeon continually controls bleeding throughout each step of the facelift. The author prefers the 4.0-mHz radiowave system (Ellman International, Oceanside, New York) to conventional electrosurgery. This system provides simultaneous incision with coagulation and produces less lateral thermal damage than conventional electrosurgery. Using a combination of

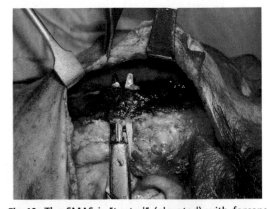

Fig. 10. The SMAS is "tented" (elevated) with forceps before incision and excision to remain superior to the parotidomasseteric fascia. This image shows the facelift scissors under the SMAS and over the parotidomasseteric fascia.

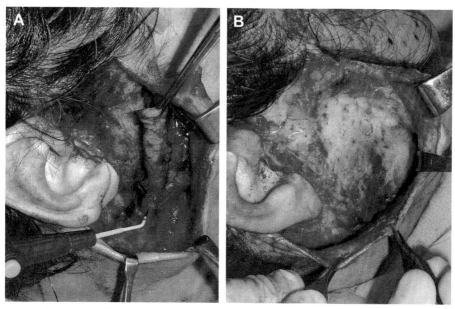

Fig. 11. The motor branches of the facial nerve are most vulnerable because they exit the parotid gland over the surface of the masseter muscle. (*A*) SMAS rectangle is shown being excised. (*B*) Exposed masseter and platysma muscles inferior to the parotidomasseteric fascia and anterior to the parotid gland are shown.

bayonet bipolar forceps (large tip and fine tip), a ball electrode, and indirect forceps coagulation allows the surgeon a multitude of means of addressing bleeding (**Fig. 14**).

In the discussion of complications, a small but significant point is to protect the delicate lipocutaneous flap from thermal insult when using electrosurgery. Because any electrosurgical coagulation can produce heat, cauterizing fat can create a heat sink that can remain extremely hot for

several seconds. It is important for the assistant not to allow the skin flap to contact the cauterized area until it is cools, because a full-thickness thermal burn can occur (**Fig. 15**).

ADDRESSING COMPLICATIONS RELATED TO SKIN PULL AND EXCISION

After the SMAS is addressed and hemostasis is achieved, the skin is the next topic of importance.

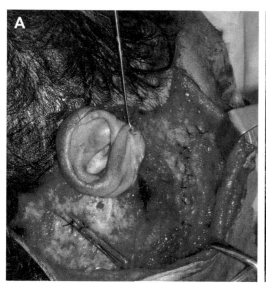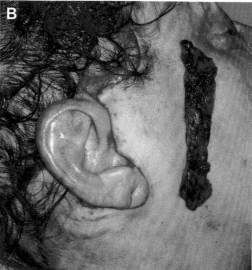

Fig. 12. SMASectomy after reapproximation of the borders with the sutures in place (*A*) and the excised SMAS overlying its approximate position (*B*).

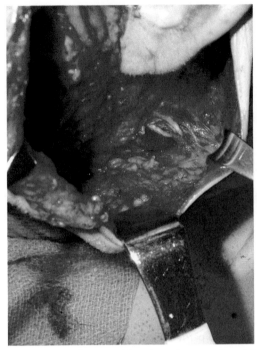

Fig. 13. GAN and external jugular vein are vulnerable to injury when dissecting over the SCM region. The image shows the left-sided external jugular vein and GAN branch.

Numerous pitfalls await the unprepared or inexperienced facelift surgeon. One of the most common problems is the control (or lack thereof) when addressing the vectors of skin pull. Although it seems obvious which vector of direction would produce the most natural result, experience shows many patients who have an unnatural or upswept appearance. When a patient says that "I don't want to look like Joan Rivers," what he or she is commenting on is the "pulled back" or "wind tunnel" look that is often a result of unnatural skin vector pull. Ideally, the incisions should be designed to pull the skin perpendicular to the incision. The

surgeon must still control the vector of pull to be natural for that specific patient, and the author personally believes that although it is a general vector, it is actually a little different for each patient. Having said this, the surgeon must deal with a combination of vertical, horizontal, and oblique vectors of tension. There is usually a "sweet spot" that produces the most esthetic vector, and the vectors of pull should be a combination of this most natural vector (**Fig. 16**). Failing to observe the optimum vector can lead to the "upswept" look. This is especially noticeable in a patient who has significant skin wrinkling (**Fig. 17**). These patients must be advised before surgery that unless they plan a resurfacing procedure before, during, or after the facelift, the facial wrinkles may be pulled in a direction that makes them more noticeable.

Another huge problem with facelift skin adjustment is an unnatural-appearing earlobe. Although this seems like a straightforward part of the lift, failure to address the earlobe properly can lead to the most telltale sign of a poor technique, which is a "pixie" earlobe (**Fig. 18**). The pixie or "elfin" earlobe is a result of lack of attention to the skin cutback to deliver the earlobe from under the excess pulled skin. The classic mistake is to overcut the skin cutback at the base of the lobe. When this happens, the lobe is sutured more inferiorly to the cheek skin. Hanging the earlobe on the cheek is never a good idea and causes an elongated pull of the lobe that can ruin the esthetics of an otherwise successful facelift. The surgeon must also keep in mind that when performing facelift surgery, the patient is supine and that when the patient is upright, gravity is going to pull on the lobe-cheek interface even more. For this reason, the adage of "measure twice, cut once" is never more applicable than here. In smaller facelifts, it should be attempted to deliver the lobe from the overlying flap without any cutting of the flap. The novice surgeon may be surprised how many times this can occur. If the lobe cannot be passively delivered from the

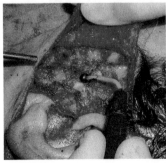
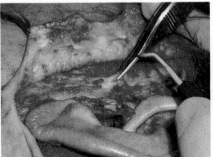
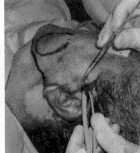

Fig. 14. There are multiple means of controlling bleeding during facelift surgery using (*left to right*) ball cautery, indirect forceps coagulation, and bipolar forceps coagulation.

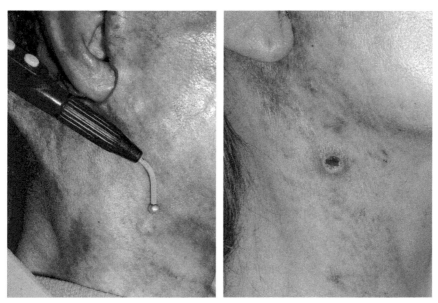

Fig. 15. Allowing the delicate lipocutaneous facelift flap to contact cauterized tissue before cooling can cause a full-thickness burn.

flap, extremely small cutbacks should be made and lobe delivery reattempted until the lobe sits tight in the crouch of the flap (**Fig. 19**). It is far better to have an earlobe that is set too high than one that is set too low and is pulled into a triangle. After the lobe is delivered, microadjustments can be made so that the lobe lies passively and is not bunched. Again, a small amount of bunching is allowable, because when the patient returns to the upright position, the cheek is going to pull the earlobe down several millimeters.

Another point worth mentioning in terms of earlobes is that fact that patients are soon going to be rolling over in bed, wearing pullover tops, placing earrings, and otherwise doing their unintentional best to disrupt your beautifully placed earlobe. Although the author closes his anterior and posterior facelift incisions with resorbable 5-0 gut suture, it is prudent to place several 4-0 Vicryl sutures at the base of the lobe to add extended support over the healing process.

High on the list of having the "done" look is an unnatural-appearing tragus (**Fig. 20**). The normal tragus is well defined and covers much of the external auditory meatus from the lateral view. Although patients do not usually notice or complain about a blunted tragus, it is quite obvious to the trained eye. One advantage of pretragal

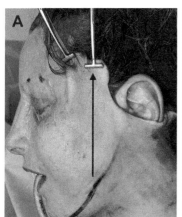
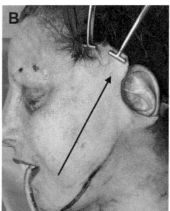
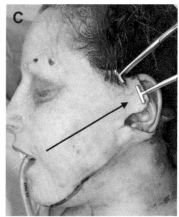

Fig. 16. Photographs illustrate the general combination of skin pull vectors in the vertical (*A*), horizontal (*B*), and oblique (*C*) directions.

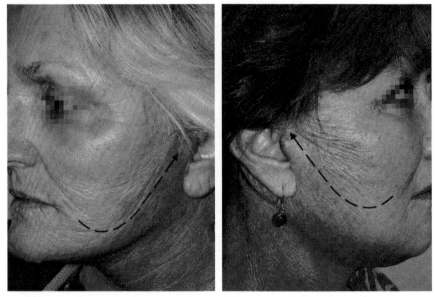

Fig. 17. Patients with extensive actinic damage or skin wrinkling can be left with unnatural appearing wrinkles if this issue is not addressed. Extreme care to vector position is necessary to prevent this upswept look, but it is sometimes impossible without some adjunctive procedure, such as carbon dioxide laser resurfacing.

incisions over posttragal incisions is that the tragus is not deformed. There is a distinct learning curve when reconstructing the tragus from the facelift flap. If the surgeon is not adept at tragal reconstruction, he or she is better off using the pretragal approach. With some practice and patience, predictable tragal esthetics are reproducible. One problem encountered in sculpting the new tragus is the mobility of that tissue, especially when using

scalpel blades. To stabilize the tragus during sculpting, the author places a 5-0 gut suture at the tragal notch above and below the tragus to stabilize the tissue (**Fig. 21**A). Once the site is stabilized, the Ellman fine-wire electrode is used to contour the stabilized tissue to its natural curvaceous nature.[21,22] The fine-wire electrode allows a "pressureless" incision, which greatly assists sculpting of mobile tissue (see **Fig. 21**B).

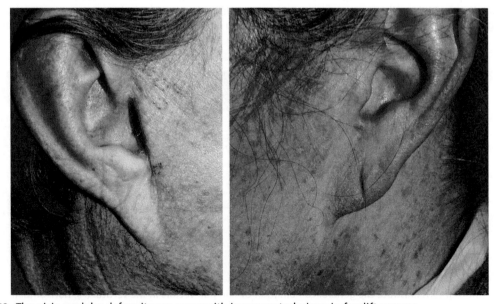

Fig. 18. The pixie ear lobe deformity can occur with improper technique in facelift surgery.

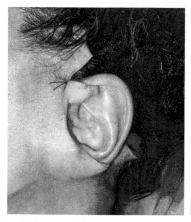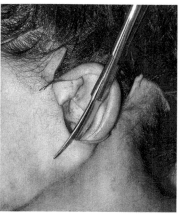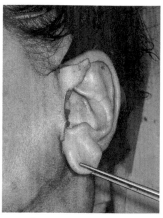

Fig. 19. It should first be attempted to pull the earlobe out of the flap without any skin cutback. If adjustment is required, skin cutbacks should be made in microadjustments to allow a passive position of the lobe after suturing. The image illustrates the steps in creating a natural-appearing earlobe.

Fig. 21C shows the sculpted tragus, and **Fig. 21**D shows the final sutures in place. It is important not to overcontour the tissue and actually to allow some excess tissue, because the area is going to contract in the postoperative period. If the skin in this area is closed with tension, the tragus is going to be retracted anteriorly, exposing the external auditory meatus.

COMPLICATIONS INVOLVING PATIENTS AFTER FACELIFT PROCEDURES

Having addressed some of the more common preoperative and intraoperative facelift complications and their prevention, the final focus of this article is on postoperative facelift complications. As somewhat addressed previously in this article, a postoperative expanding hematoma is a true emergency in facelift surgery.[23–26] An expanding hematoma puts the delicate lipocutaneous flap under significant pressure and can compromise the dermal plexus and other vascular nourishment of the flap. This can result in minor or major loss of flap viability, with resultant skin necrosis and full-thickness scarring. The points of prevention were addressed previously, but when an expanding hematoma does occur (and the statistics range from 2%–15% of hematomas doing so), the surgeon must be able to diagnose and treat the complication rapidly to divert tissue loss.[27]

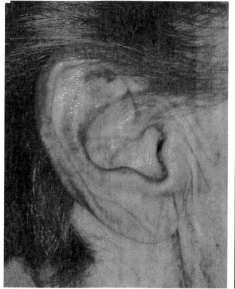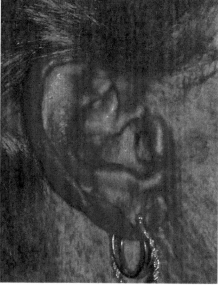

Fig. 20. Blunted or otherwise unnatural-appearing tragi are stigmata of poor surgical technique.

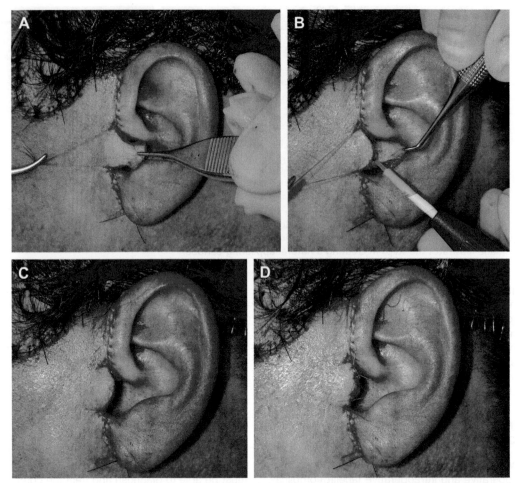

Fig. 21. (*A*) Excess tissue secured with two sutures to stabilize the mobile tissue. (*B*) Fine-wire radiowave surgery electrode sculpting and thinning of the tissue. (*C*) Sculpted tragus passively in place. (*D*) Final tragal anatomy.

Postoperative bleeding with a hematoma can (and does) result immediately at the end of the case and is noticed when washing the hair or bandaging the patient. Every attempt should be made at that time to evacuate and control the bleeding. Because the surgeon is frequently out of the operating suite at this time, the staff must be well trained in recognizing problematic bleeding. Fortunately, this early "on the table" accumulation of blood responds to evacuation with a small blunt liposuction cannula (or needle aspiration) and light compression (**Fig. 22**). The blood is suctioned, and compression of the pre- and postauricular flaps is performed with small stacks of 4×4 gauze. The area is checked again after 10 minutes for reaccumulation. If there is reaccumulation, the evacuation and pressure can be repeated again, but continued accumulation is grounds for opening the incision and exploring and controlling the bleeding, especially if the accumulation is bright red blood.

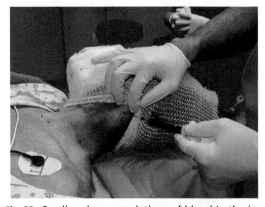

Fig. 22. Small early accumulations of blood in the immediate postoperative period can frequently be evacuated and controlled with pressure before bandaging. Continued accumulation warrants exploration and control of the source.

Postoperative hematomas can be categorized into minor and major categories. A minor accumulation of blood can be evacuated the next day or is oftentimes resorbed. A major hematoma expanding in real time is emergent. Because these frequently occur in the early postoperative period, it makes sense to recover the patient in your facility for several hours. Having said this, the next 24 hours still present a vulnerable period, and checking on the patient throughout the evening is time well spent. Also, educating the patient on the signs and symptoms of expanding hematoma can increase the chances of early treatment. During the past decade, the author has personally had four cases of major expanding hematomas that required emergent treatment. Two of these, although significantly distorting the patient's face, were not recognized by the patient or family and were seen at the next morning's postoperative visit (**Fig. 23**). One of these was unilateral, and the other was bilateral. The other two patients called within 8 hours of their facelift, reporting severe unilateral pain; they were noticeably agitated and reported rapid onset swelling with bleeding from the incision sites (**Fig. 24**). One of these patients also reported that it was difficult to close her mouth.

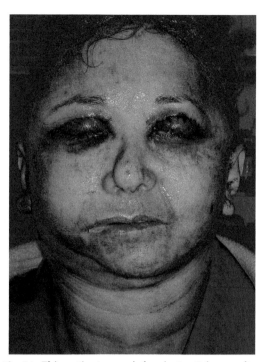

Fig. 24. This patient paged the doctor 8 hours after surgery and complained of intense right-sided pain and inability to close her mouth, and she was noticeably agitated. She presented with an obvious right-sided expanding hematoma and was taken back to surgery.

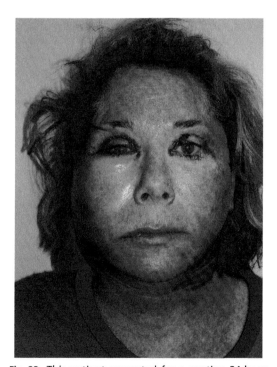

Fig. 23. This patient presented for a routine 24-hour follow-up and was unaware that any problem existed. Unlike most patients with a hematoma, she denied severe pain or agitation. She reported a coughing spell in the middle of the night followed by "some swelling".

This resulted from dissection of blood into the buccal space, which expanded between the upper and lower teeth.

All these patients were treated in the same successful manner, although none of them were treated conveniently. Treatment of a major expanding hematoma requires removing the sutures and opening the flaps to explore for the bleeder(s). Generally, these patients are scared, agitated, and in pain, and treatment is difficult without intravenous sedation. Once the flaps are opened, large "currant jelly" clots are observed and debrided with gauze and a large-bore liposuction cannula (**Figs. 25** and **26**). The operative sites are then irrigated with saline to assist in identification of the source or sources of bleeding. The author believe that the accumulation of a large clot acts as an irritant to the underlying tissue and frequently causes multiple bleeding sites other than the actual offending vessel. Generally, these areas of irritation-induced bleeding are easily controlled; however, finding the exact offending vessel can sometimes be difficult. In some cases, the surgeon finds that the offending bleeder is a venous or arterial vessel that was previously cauterized and has ruptured. Other cases present with a bleeder

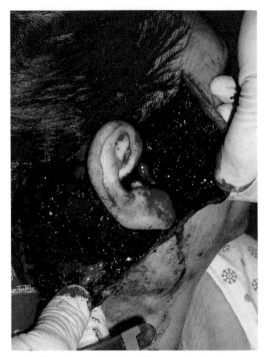

Fig. 25. The "currant jelly" clot is visualized after opening the surgical site.

that was hidden under the flap or simply overlooked. The author has never seen a sub-SMAS bleeder that caused a hematoma, and the offending vessel is usually identified. In resistant cases, it helps to pack the flaps with chilled saline gauze and apply pressure for several minutes before re-exploring. In some cases, it can be a vessel on the dermal side of the flap or a deeper large vessel, such as a superficial temporal vessel, which is pierced with a suture needle later in the latter case (**Fig. 27**). Once the bleeding is controlled,

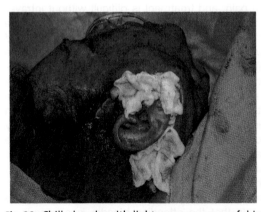

Fig. 26. Chilled packs with light pressure are useful in assisting in hemostasis during the treatment of a hematoma.

the incisions are resutured. The flap and incisions heal after being reopened and manipulated. In the hematomas that the author has treated, the offending side has always healed without complication (**Fig. 28**).

Minor hematomas or seromas can also occur after surgery because of breakdown of clotted blood and general tissue response to injury. These may occur early or up to several weeks after surgery. They are easily aspirated with an 18-gauge needle (**Fig. 29**). It is not uncommon for these to reoccur and require aspiration multiple times until they resolve. These minor seromas do not routinely jeopardize flap viability.

Other postoperative facelift complications that are commonly seen include edema and ecchymosis. Although all patients undergoing a facelift procedure experience some degree of postsurgical edema, some patients exhibit impressive swelling. Patients undergoing multiple procedures, including brow lift, midface implants, lip implants, and simultaneous laser resurfacing, can swell to alarming proportions (**Fig. 30**). Although this usually does not present significant problems, it could cause excess tension on the suture lines. The biggest problem is generally the fear of the patient and family that something bad has happened. Treatment with oral steroids usually hastens the resolution of the severe edema; however, some patients take longer than others. At the time of the consent process, patients undergoing multiple procedures and their families must be made aware of the possibility of severe edema.

Ecchymosis is another aspect of the consent process that should be discussed before surgery. Of all the precision with which experienced surgeons can explain procedures to patients, edema and ecchymosis remain the most difficult to predict. The author sees patients who predict that they are going to bruise severely and they heal without any ecchymosis, whereas some young and healthy patients sometimes bruise remarkably (**Fig. 31**).

The author believes that the standard of care is to obtain coagulation studies on patients undergoing a facelift, although there is rarely a correlation to ecchymosis. Avoiding all the common medications, herbs, and homeopathic preparations that may affect platelet function is pretty basic and well known to all surgeons. In the author's anecdotal experience, pretunneling the facelift flaps with a blunt cannula before scissors dissection has seemed to reduce ecchymosis. For years, the author has had colleagues who advocated an Arnica Montana regimen (SinEcch; Alpine Pharmaceuticals, San Rafael, California) during the pre- and postoperative periods, and he was never

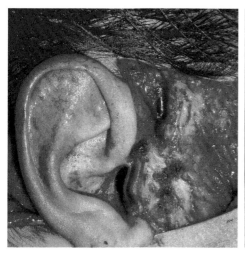
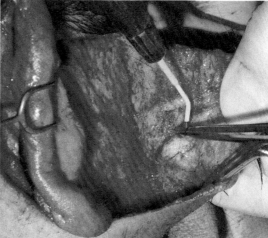

Fig. 27. Superficial temporal vein or other deep large vessels can be damaged during surgery and bleed. The underside of the lipocutaneous flap can contain smaller vessels capable of causing an expanding hematoma and should not be overlooked.

convinced of its effectiveness. After trying this on a consecutive number of patients, he has changed his thought process, because, in fact, it seems to make a difference, although he cannot back that claim up statistically.

Two of the most feared complications of facelift surgery are motor and sensory nerve damage and flap necrosis.[28] These, unlike many of the complications discussed previously, can be tragic for the patient and surgeon and can lead to damage of reputation and litigation.

Patients undergoing facelift procedures must be educated in the fact that they are all going to have some component of sensory deficit, especially in the pre- and postauricular regions. Generally, this sensory deficit spontaneously resolves over a 90-day period. They must be reassured when it takes longer, and reinnervation usually ensues with time. Some discussion of motor nerve deficit has been discussed previously. Frontal, buccal, zygomatic, marginal mandibular, and cervical nerve injury can be caused by many different things, including direct injury (clamps, needles, scalpels, and scissors); neurapraxia (stretching from overaggressive retraction); thermal injury from cautery; compression injury from sutures, edema, or hematoma;

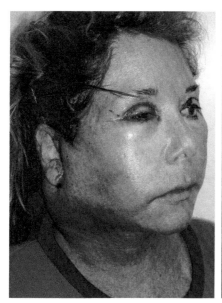
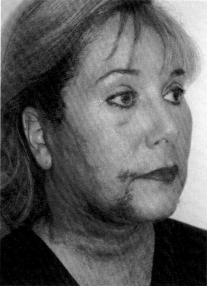

Fig. 28. Patient in **Fig. 21** is shown 8 days after treating the hematoma and resuturing the surgical site.

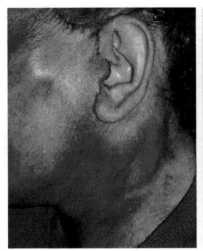
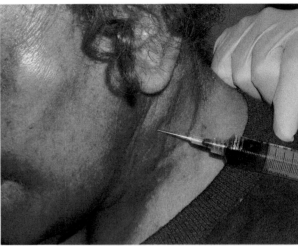

Fig. 29. Seromas can occur early or later in the postoperative healing phase and are easily treated by simple aspiration. This patient is shown with a minor seroma 1 week after surgery, which was aspirated with an 18-gauge needle.

and other causes. This is disconcerting for the patient and surgeon in the early postoperative period, but most of these conditions spontaneously resolve within weeks or months. A gradual return of function to the affected area is seen and greeted with comfort by all involved. Patients should be reassured that the nerve weakness is likely temporary, but they should be advised (before surgery) that return of full function cannot be guaranteed. In the hundreds of facelifts that the author has performed over the past 12 years, he has experienced no permanent motor nerve injuries. He has experienced four to five patients who had unilateral paresis of the buccal, zygomatic, or marginal mandibular branches with altered animation that returned within 90 to 120 days (**Fig. 32**). Motor nerve injuries that do not seem to improve or those that are severe and include multiple nerve branches should be evaluated by a surgeon experienced in microneurosurgery after 90 days.

Necrosis of the lipocutaneous flap can lead to permanent scars and extended recovery. Causes

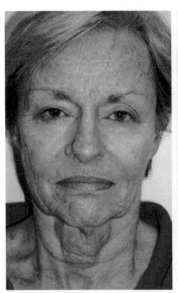
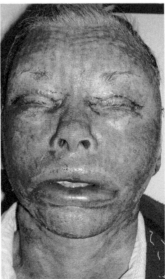
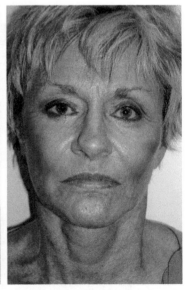

Fig. 30. This patient is shown before, 24 hours after, and 30 days after multiple facial procedures, including rhytidectomy, midface implants, lip implants, upper and lower eyelid surgery, and laser resurfacing. Multiple combined procedures can cause extreme swelling in some patients.

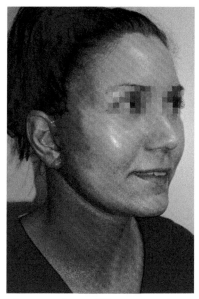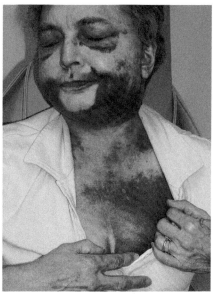

Fig. 31. Both patients are shown 48 hours after the same facelift procedure, and the differences in individual propensity for bruising are illustrated.

vary from bandage compression, patient sleeping position, flap sutures under tension, inherent healing problems, and no discernible cause. Although it is more common in smokers or patients with compromised health, it can happen in the best of circumstances. Fortunately, the posterior auricular region is the most prone area to flap breakdown and is generally out of sight of the patient and can be covered by hairstyle. Although these areas of nonviable tissue appear extremely angry and inflamed in the initial phases, they generally heal with minor scarring (**Fig. 33**). Tissue death on the preauricular or visible anterior facial skin can be much more problematic because it can be severe and leave permanent scars that may require skin grafts. Small areas (the size of a quarter) generally scab over and regranulate from the base. Some practitioners recommend topical application of

nitroglycerin paste to encourage local vasodilation. Interim treatment with antibiotics and wound care usually produces an acceptable scar that can be improved with carbon dioxide laser resurfacing. For large areas of flap necrosis, emergent efforts, such as hyperbaric oxygen therapy, may be necessary in addition to consultation with a practitioner versed in wound care.

Postsurgical Revision

The best intentions of the surgeon are sometimes not met for numerous reasons and can leave the patient and surgeon with a suboptimal result. Sometimes, because of patient variability or extreme skin excess and ptosis, the result is as good as it reasonably can be. Educating the patient on such matters at the consent process can

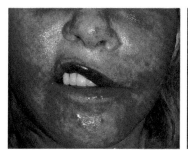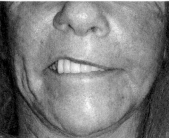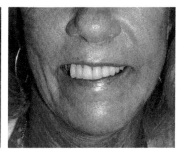

Fig. 32. Patient is shown with facial nerve paresis of the left-sided buccal and zygomatic facial nerve branches. She is shown at 1 week, 2 months, and 3 months after surgery. Her improvement at 90 days is consistent with this type of minor nerve injury.

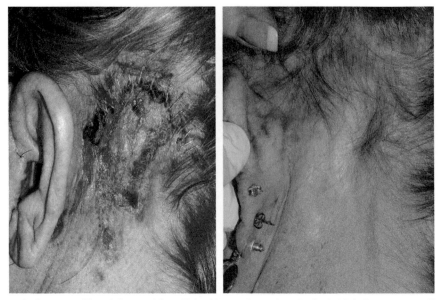

Fig. 33. Postauricular wound breakdown, although looking quite serious in the initial phases, generally heals with acceptable results with simple wound care. The patient is shown at 10 days and 5 months after facelift surgery with posterior auricular wound breakdown. The patient was a smoker and was aware of this possible complication before surgery.

head off ill feelings. An example is a patient with a short thick neck and a low- and anterior-sitting hyoid bone. These patients have extremely oblique cervicomental angles and, in the best of circumstances (even with aggressive submentoplasty), are never going to have a "90° neck" (**Fig. 34**). Underpromising with significant preoperative examination and discussion can mitigate some of these postoperative points of contention.

Prudent postoperative patient education is paramount to avoid patient-generated complications. Although heat may be beneficial for edema occurring after a facelift, the skin is frequently insensate

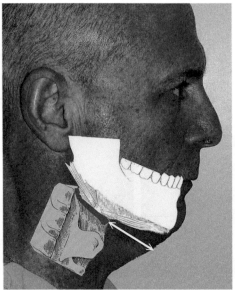
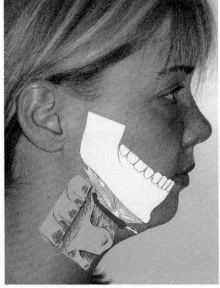

Fig. 34. The author keeps this diagram in each evaluation room and shows problematic patients why their inherent neck and submental anatomy may compromise their postoperative neck esthetics in severe situations.

in the initial recovery period and patients can sustain severe burns from heating pads,[29] hot-water bottles, chemical thermal heating devices, and curling irons or hair driers (**Fig. 35**). All patients need a list of these potential pitfalls that could affect the surgeon's work and their results.

Other postoperative situations exist in which the patient was simply undertreated (or sometimes overtreated) and requires revision. The author generally performs reasonable revisions free of charge in the first year after facelift surgery, especially if they are of his doing. If they represent situations that were not necessarily reflective of his work, he may charge a reasonable materials or anesthesia fee. Although there is no implied warranty with cosmetic surgery, it is a consumer-driven market, and if the author purchased a wide-screen television for $5000 and it did not function properly, he would expect a repair or replacement. That is just good basic customer service, and, again, we are in the customer service business. On a selfish note, the author also does not want any patient walking around with a suboptimal result that is credited to his work. A cosmetic surgeon's results and reputation are everything.

ODDS AND ENDS

A facelift procedure (often with multiple other cosmetic procedures) is a big deal, and it takes some time for the "smoke to clear" for the true final result. Along the healing process, there are many small things that bother the patient (or surgeon). Hypertrophic surgical scars, palpable lumps under the skin, irregularities on the posterior auricular surface, transient hair loss, pigmentation abnormalities, lingering edema, and asymmetry represent some of these situations. Explaining to the patient that these are common and treating the patient free of charge can go a long way toward patient relations. It is not unusual to inject a steroid

in hypertrophic scars, smooth out bumps behind the ear, or address these other issues along the way. In a busy facelift practice, someone is always on the mend and addressing these small problems is as much a part of the process as in the scenario of a painter who must return to a home to touch up small imperfections. Letting patients know this up front puts them at ease when these small issues present.

INFORMED CONSENT PROCESS

Paramount to everything discussed in this article is adequate preoperative informed consent and education for the patients. Although our offices perform these procedures weekly, we must keep in mind that it is foreign for our patients and they frequently have a "television mentality" that surgery and healing occur rapidly and without incident. A patient cannot be overeducated about a procedure. Some patients do not understand as well as others, and some preoperative time is well spent to prevent a problematic patient. Patients must understand what is normal and what is not, what is a sequela, and what is a complication. They must understand the entire process of what happens when there is a problem, who is going to fix it, and who is going to bear the cost, for example. They must understand that their role in pre- and postoperative care can have a dramatic impact on the final result and that the surgeon is not alone in this.

The author also uses supplementary consent forms to stress points that may require additional emphasis. He uses a "smoker's consent" form to underline the problematic nature of facelift surgery in that patient group. He also has a consent form entitled "what your facelift won't do." This details such things as the fact that as "a facelift is not an operation for wrinkles," "a facelift won't improve your eyes or brow," "a facelift will not

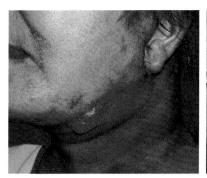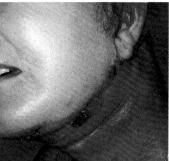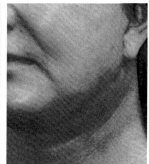

Fig. 35. Because of the lack of normal sensation in the early postoperative period, patients may injure themselves. This patient used a heating pad and sustained a significant burn that, fortunately, healed with minimal scarring.

make your nasolabial folds disappear," or "you may need a touch up of your facelift" in addition to other details that patients may misunderstand in the procedure, recovery, and result.

SUMMARY

It is impossible to detail all facets of possible facelift complications in an 8500-word article, because they could fill volumes of texts. There are many less common complications that were not covered in this article, such as parotid fistula, scar revision, infection, and wound dehiscence, for example. There exist many well-written texts and journal articles to assist the surgeon with the management of the less frequently seen complications, and in this day and age of the Internet, they are only a click away. Fortunately, severe complications with facelift surgery are rare. Most complications are predictable in occurrence and treatment, and the average surgeon who is competent enough to perform a facelift properly is also usually competent enough to manage the common complications. A surgeon who does not have complications is a surgeon who does not operate much. A surgeon who has repeated complications may be in need of enlightenment. Complications are always a part of surgery, and preparing for them in advance, understanding their mechanism of occurrence, and having the knowledge and experience to treat them are requirements for being good at what you do.

REFERENCES

1. Lexer E. Zur gesichtsplastik. Arch Klin Chir 1910;92: 749.
2. Joseph J. Plastic operation on protruding cheek. Dtsch Med Wochenschr 1921;47:287.
3. Joseph J. Nasenplastikand sonstige gesichtsplastik negsteinen anhang tiber mammaplastic. Leipaig Curt Kabitzach 1928;525–7.
4. Joseph J. Verbesserung meiner hangemangenplastic (melomioplastic). Dtsch Med Wochenschr 1928;54:567.
5. Passot R. La cheirurgie esthetique des rides du visage. Presse Med 1919;27:258.
6. Passot R. La xhirurgie esthetique pure (technique et resultants). Paris: Gaston Doin Cie; 1931. p. 176–80.
7. Morestin H. La reduction graduelle des deformities tegumentaries. Bull Mem Soc Chir Paris 1915;41:1233.
8. Brouguet J. La xhirurgie esthetique de la face. Concours Med 1921;1657–70.
9. Lagarde M. Nouvelles techniques pour le traitement des rides de la face et de cou. Arch Franco-Belg Chir 1928;31:1954.
10. Noel A. La chirurgie estique son role social. Paris: Mason Cie; 1926. p. 62–6.
11. Noel A. La chirurgie esthetique. Clearmont (Oise): Thiron et Cie; 1928.
12. Skoog T. Plastic surgery: new methods and refinements. Philadelphia: WB Saunders; 1975.
13. Mitz V, Peyronie M. The superficial musculoaponeurotic system (SMAS) in the parotid and cheek area. Plast Reconstr Surg 1976;58:80–8.
14. Antell DE, Orseck MJ. A comparison of face lift techniques in eight consecutive sets of identical twins. Plast Reconstr Surg 2007;120(6):1667–73.
15. Adamson JC, Horton CE, Crawford HH. The surgical correction of the "turkey gobbler" deformity. Plast Reconstr Surg 1964;34:598.
16. Rees TD, Aston S. Clinical evaluation of submuscu-loaponeurotic dissection and fixation in facelift surgery. Plast Reconstr Surg 1977;60:859–61.
17. Webster RC, Smith RC, Papsidero MJ, et al. Comparison of SMAS plication with SMAS imbrication in face lifting. Laryngoscope 1982;92(8 Pt 1): 901–12.
18. Baker DC. Minimal incision rhytidectomy (short scar facelift) with lateral SMASectomy: evolution and application. Aesthetic Surg J 2001;21:14–26.
19. Hamara ST. Composite rhytidectomy. St, Louis (MO): Quality Publilshing; 1993.
20. Baker DC. Lateral SMASectomy. Plast Reconstr Surg 1997;100(2):509–13.
21. Niamtu J. 4.0 MHz radiowave surgery in cosmetic surgery. Australasian Journal of Cosmetic Surgery 2005;1(1):52–9.
22. Niamtu J. 4.0 MHz radiowave surgery in cosmetic facial surgery. In: Bell WH, Guerroro CA, editors. Distraction osteogenesis of the facial skeleton. Ontario, Canada: BC Decker; 2007. p. 30–7.
23. Baker D. Rhytidectomy with lateral SMASectomy. Facial Plast Surg 2000;16(3):209–13.
24. Rees TD, Aston SJ. Complications of rhytidectomy. Clin Plast Surg 1978;5(1):109–19.
25. Baker DC. Complications of cervicofacial rhytidectomy. Clin Plast Surg 1983;10(3):543–62.
26. Griffin JE, Jo C. Complications after superficial plane cervicofacial rhytidectomy: a retrospective analysis of 178 consecutive facelifts and review of the literature. J Oral Maxillofac Surg 2007;65(11): 2227–34.
27. Niamtu J. Expanding hematoma in face-lift surgery: literature review, case presentations, and caveats. Dermatol Surg 2005;31:1134–44.
28. Baker DC, Conley J. Avoiding facial nerve injuries in rhytidectomy. Anatomical variations and pitfalls. Plast Reconstr Surg 1979;64(6):781–95.
29. Dini GM, Ferreira LM. Burns due to heating pads. Plast Reconstr Surg 2007;120(7):2126–7.

Complications of Rhinoplasty

Brian C. Harsha, DDS, MS

KEYWORDS

- Rhinoplasty • Complications • Cosmetic surgery

Rhinoplasty is generally considered one of the most difficult cosmetic operative procedures performed today. It requires a three-dimensional manipulation of various tissues, often performed with limited access. Results in rhinoplasty can depend on the doctor's surgical skill and variations in the patient's skin thickness, subcutaneous tissue, cartilage, bone, and mucous membranes. The surgeon must develop an effective method to reliably and predictably alter and sculpture the elements of the nose. Typically, a graduated or systematic process should be developed to produce the desired result based on the existing anatomy of the patient. No standard rhinoplasty operation exists, because the underlying anatomy of each patient is unique. Therefore, surgeons must develop not only the ability to analyze the anatomic relationships of the nasal structures but also techniques to adequately alter these structures for each patient's anatomy. No single incision, approach, or manipulation of the tissues can be used in every case. Through years of experience and meticulous record-keeping, surgeons can develop predictable and reliable results, which will minimize the need for revision surgery. The final result of surgery is a combination of the surgical manipulation of the tissues and the healing responses of multiple different tissue types. However, the final result is often not visualized until years after the procedure is performed. A result that looks perfect 1 week postoperatively may seem overly operated 1 year later.

The literature reports an incidence of postoperative rhinoplasty complications ranging from 5% to 28%.[1–4] Minor irregularities may only be appreciated by the surgeon and not require reoperation. However, results considered by the surgeon to be perfectly may be viewed as a failure by the patient.

Many factors may influence the final outcome in rhinoplasty. Skin thickness can be a blessing and a curse. Patients who have thick skin can undergo extensive alterations to the underlying cartilaginous and bony structures without fear of the appearance of minor irregularities. Unfortunately, thicker skin will not redrape as well, and a refined nose may not be possible to produce. Conversely, thin skin can easily display the surgeons' skill for manipulating underlying tissues. Unfortunately, minor irregularities in the shape and symmetry of the underlying tissues will also be easily visible. Patients older than 40 years have their own unique anatomic considerations. Elderly patients' skin becomes increasingly inelastic and therefore less able to redrape properly postsurgically. The cartilage may be calcified, and the bones of the nose and septum tend to be more brittle. Finally, decreased vascularity of the tissues may also affect surgical outcome.

Generally, complications in rhinoplasty can be divided into those that occur early and those that tend to occur or become apparent late in the postoperative period. Early complications can include hemorrhage, hematoma, infection, periostitis, edema, ecchymosis, skin problems, and septal perforations. Many of these complications in rhinoplasty can be avoided through meticulous attention to detail during the operative procedure, and is perhaps most important at the end of the operative procedure. A final check of the surgical result before suturing and splinting is mandatory. The bony and cartilaginous dorsum should be inspected for small spicules of bone or cartilage and minor irregularities. Rubbing a moistened finger over the dorsum can help identify any areas that need final adjustment. The skin envelope is examined to make sure no small pieces of debris

Coastal Facial Aesthetic & Laser Surgery, 708 21st Avenue North, Myrtle Beach, SC 29577, USA
E-mail address: bharsha@sc.rr.com

Oral Maxillofacial Surg Clin N Am 21 (2009) 81–89
doi:10.1016/j.coms.2008.10.005
1042-3699/08/$ – see front matter © 2009 Elsevier Inc. All rights reserved.

remain that could contribute to infection or visible irregularities. Wound edges are then gently approximated to provide ideal healing. Taping and splinting are used to stabilize and maintain surgical manipulations.

Late complications generally involve abnormalities of the nasal tip, cartilaginous vault, and bony vault. They usually involve either over- or underresection or asymmetrical resection of the involved tissues. These complications may occur because of a failure to understand the consequences of surgical manipulation of the tissues, or from the idiosyncrasies of the various anatomic tissues' healing.

EARLY COMPLICATIONS
Hemorrhage

Hemorrhage or epistaxis usually occurs either during the first 48 hours or at 10 to 14 days postoperatively. Patients must undergo preoperative screening for any medications that may interfere with normal clotting or make the patient prone to postoperative bleeding. Aspirin and salicylates are generally discontinued 10 to 14 days before surgery. Patients should be specifically asked about herbal medications, because they often do not consider these "real medicine." Patients undergoing rhinoplasty should generally be normotensive pre- and postoperatively. Bleeding may be encountered from raw edges of the cartilaginous incisions. Bleeding is most likely to occur at the transfixion incision or anterior septal mucosal incisions. Proper closure of these incisions at surgery will minimize this complication.

The second most common time for postoperative bleeding occurs from the 10th to 14th day, most likely because the maturing clot separates from the incision. If the bleeding occurs from the anterior nose, the exact point should be identified and treated using direct vision. Severe bleeding may require anterior and posterior nasal packs. Persistent bleeding may rarely require hospitalization and treatment in the operating room.

Hematoma

Bleeding underneath the skin flap may cause displacement and distortion of the nasal tissues. Thick amounts of clotted blood underneath the skin can produce excessive scar tissue and disruption of the normal healing mechanisms. Hematomas of the dorsal skin can also be produced during removal of the cast. Great care should be taken to adequately loosen any plaster or tape from the skin before its removal. Mild soap or orange solvent applied to cotton applicators can be used to soften plaster and Steri-Strips. Septal hematomas can cause nasal obstruction and septal perforations if not treated promptly. Patients undergoing submucous resection or other septal procedures typically have a light nasal packing placed to help hemostasis (**Fig. 1**). Careful inspection of these areas for a hematoma is mandatory.

Infection

Infection after rhinoplasty is generally much less common than might be anticipated. Rhinoplasty is generally performed after a nasal prep but considered an unsterile operation. Antibiotics are typically used in the perioperative period. Typically a broad-spectrum cephalosporin can be used for antibiotic prophylaxis. Small localized abscesses can occur along the incision lines or in areas where surgical debris has collected, and can be treated with incision and drainage along with the appropriate antibiotics. Typically, these infections are caused by *Staphylococcus aureus* or, rarely, a Pseudomonas infection. A minor low-grade infection may occur along the osteotomy sites as a result of bone dust left behind. Pain, swelling, and erythema may be present. Initial treatment consists of antibiotic therapy. If the infection persist, drainage of the area and removal of any debris or sequestrum may be necessary (**Fig. 2**).

Toxic shock syndrome has been reported in cases of nasal packing. The proximity of the

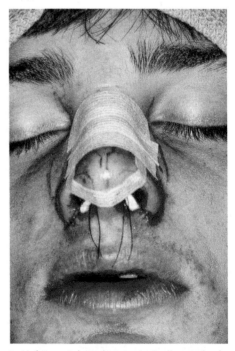

Fig. 1. Light septal packs are typically used when a septoplasty is performed.

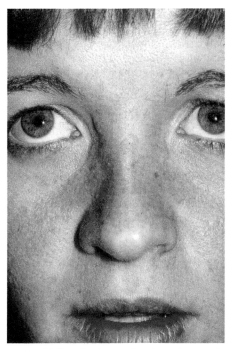

Fig. 2. A small chronic abscess developed along the superior aspect of the right lateral osteotomy. Antibiotics did not resolve it and a small incision with curettage was required.

cavernous sinus makes basal meningitis possible, although fortunately rare.[5]

Edema and Ecchymosis

Swelling after rhinoplasty is an expected result and therefore not a true complication. However, the amount of swelling is greatly variable among patients. Some surgeons believe using perioperative glucocorticoid steroids helps reduce edema, although definitive clinical studies have not been produced. For most patients, most swelling in the nasal tip and nasal dorsum resolve and the final result visualized after 6 to 12 months. Small changes in the nasal tip may be seen as late as 2 years postoperatively. If the occurrence of a super tip prominence is believed to be persistent swelling, injection of steroids into the pollybeak may be helpful.

Patients who undergo lateral osteotomies are at risk for periorbital ecchymosis, which may last for 2 to 4 weeks after surgery. The use of a smaller unguarded osteotome may lower the occurrence of this complication.[6]

Skin Abnormalities

Minor skin reactions to the tape and splint may cause inflammation. Patients who have oily skin may develop pustules, although these generally resolve once the offending agent is removed. Occasionally, new spider veins or telangiectasias may develop, and excessive use of steroid injections to resolve postoperative edema may make this occurrence more common.

Skin necrosis may occur over the nasal dorsum or nasal tip. Necrosis of the dorsum skin is most likely a result of excessive pressure from the splint. If open rhinoplasty is performed simultaneously with excessive nasal lobule narrowing, vascular compromise of the nasal tip skin is possible. Weir procedures should be delayed to a secondary surgery if this is a concern.

Poor scars from the external approach are also possible. Generally the transcolumellar incision heals with an imperceptible scar. Occasionally, a more obvious scar may develop as a result of inadequate reapproximation or poor healing. Great care should be taken not to infringe on the soft tissue facets of the nasal rim when any marginal rim incision is made. Soft tissue notching can result (**Fig. 3**).

Septal Perforations

Septal hematomas that are not properly drained may lead to septal perforations. Other causes of perforations include infection, pressure necrosis, and symmetric septal mucosal tears. Small perforations may heal sufficiently through wound contraction. Keeping the area clean with hydrogen peroxide and antibiotic ointment is important. Larger perforations can be extremely difficult to close and may require large septal flaps to be elevated.

LATE COMPLICATIONS
Nasal Tip

The nasal tip may be the area that requires the most revision in rhinoplasty surgery.

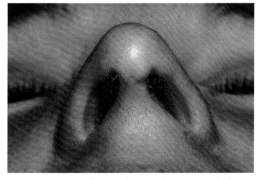

Fig. 3. Notching of the left nostril is produced by encroachment of the marginal rim incision on the soft triangle of the nostril.

Complications may result from over- or underreduction of the tip and asymmetrical resection. Rhinoplasty is a compromise, and the most conservative surgery that accomplishes the desired result is typically the best. To produce an attractive tip, clinicians must understand and maintain the support mechanisms of the nasal tip. Support mechanisms have generally been divided into two categories: major and minor. Major support mechanisms generally include: the medial and lateral crura, the medial crural footplate attachment to the caudal margin of the septal cartilage, and the attachment of the upper lateral cartilage to the lower lateral cartilage. Several minor nasal tip support mechanisms are also present: the connective tissue between the domes of the lower lateral cartilages, the cartilaginous septal dorsum, the connective tissue complex from the lateral crura to the pyriform aperture, the attachment of the lower lateral cartilages to the overlying skin, the nasal spine, and the membranous septum. Failure to preserve or reconstitute the tip support mechanism may lead to loss of vital tip support.

Overreduction of the Nasal Tip

Overresection of the lateral crus is perhaps the most common problem seen after rhinoplasty.[7] Overreduction of the lateral crus may lead to the predictable changes of alar retraction, pinching, bossing, and tip asymmetry. Overly aggressive nasal tip surgery not only results in an increase in postoperative complications but can also lead to functional disorders of the nose.[8] Many complications of nasal tip surgery arise from the operator's desire to accomplish more than is possible with the nasal tip tissues. Thick oily skin with sebaceous glands can lead to overzealous resection of the cartilaginous tip elements in an effort to produce refinement. After rhinoplasty, the tip with preexisting adequate support may appear overreduced if the tip loses further support mechanisms. In these cases, as many as possible of the major and minor tip support mechanisms should be maintained and augmenting tip support considered.

Surgical repair of the overly resected tip may require autogenous cartilage grafts to replace missing tissue. In some cases, adequate lateral crura may seem to remain, but that secondary scar contracture has overpowered the rim cartilage. Generally leaving least 6 to 9 mm of the lateral crus behind is wise. Thin-skinned individuals who possess large firm and thick alar cartilages may undergo buckling of these cartilages months or even years after the initial operation. Taking

a conservative approach is important when performing the cephalic resection of the lower lateral cartilage. Knuckling or bossae formation may also occur when interrupted strip techniques are used in thin-skinned individuals. Nasal tip onlay grafts and supportive columellar struts may improve projection in minor cases.

If severe alar retraction occurs or the ala collapse on inspiration, alar batten grafts may used for repair.[9] Severe cases may require auricular composite grafts.[10] Composite grafts can replace the missing volume and provide support to hold the nostril rim in a more anatomic position. Nasal obstruction may also occur if the upper or lower lateral cartilages prolapse into the nasal valve region. Collapse of the upper lateral cartilage is usually treated by placing a spreader graft secured between the dorsal septum and the upper lateral cartilages.

Underreduction of the Nasal Tip

Underreduction of the nasal tip structures is usually a result of inadequate attempts to produce nasal refinement.[11] However, inadequate reduction of the tip structures is preferable to overly aggressive treatment. Inadequate reduction rarely causes functional disorders that overly aggressive surgery may cause. Furthermore, because additional tip refinement is required, these complications are generally easier to correct than those associated with overly aggressive treatment. Repair of these complications usually requires exposure and delivery of the lower lateral cartilage, and is performed using the most conservative procedure that will produce the desired result. If possible, complete strip techniques are preferable (**Fig. 4**) because they offer the following advantages: preservation of tip support and projection, resistance to rotation, resistance to tip retrodisplacement, prevention of alar retraction, symmetric healing, safety, and predictability.[12] Interrupted strip techniques are reserved for patients who require maximal tip rotation, refinement, or decreased projection and who have thick skin.

Underreduction of the nasal tip may be a result of inadequate volume reduction, and is usually caused by an inadequate or unequal refinement of the alar cartilages. This effect may be caused by leaving alar cartilages behind that remain too broad. Correction would involve an approach to narrow the residual alar cartilage remnants to refine the alar cartilages.

Underresection of the nasal tip may also result in a boxy tip. In this case, the initial procedure has failed to attenuate the broad arch and spring of the alar cartilage. Again, performing a stepwise

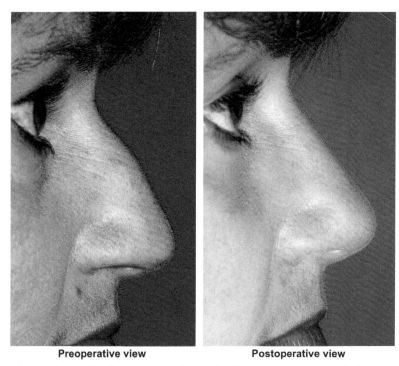

Preoperative view   **Postoperative view**

Fig. 4. Adequate tip rotation and refinement was obtained with a complete strip technique.

correction of these deformities is best. The most conservative procedure is used to produce the desire effect. Interdomal suturing, transdomal suturing, or strip interruption techniques may be necessary to weaken the spring of the lower lateral cartilage.

Underresection of an overly projected tip may also require additional correction. If the nasal tip remains overprojected after the initial surgery, repair may involve intentional disruption of the tip support mechanisms. This procedure may allow posterior retrodisplacement of the tip. Again a graduated approach can be used until the proper amount of retrodisplacement is performed. Retrodisplacement can be encouraged through complete transfixion incision, interruption and repair of the medial crura, interruption and repair of the lateral crura,[4] and dissection and reduction of the anterior nasal spine (**Fig. 5**).

Inadequate nasal tip reduction may also result in failure to rotate the nasal tip. Loss of tip support can lead to tip ptosis and the appearance of an elongated nose. Failure to adequately rotate the tip requires additional surgical procedures to produce tip rotation. Procedures that produced tip rotation include shortening of the caudal septum, columellar struts, augmentation of the nasal labial angle, or resection of a triangular piece of cartilaginous septum through a high transfixion incision.

Finally, an excessively wide alar flair may exist postoperatively, and is most common after intentional reduction of an overprojected tip. Correction includes alar base reduction. The shape of the nostril width is reduced through excision of a portion of the nostril floor and sill.

Cartilaginous Vault

Overreduction of the cartilaginous fault can result in a saddle deformity of the nasal dorsum and produce a poor supratip relationship. Careful evaluation during the initial surgery may lessen the chances of this deformity. If the surgeon notes that excessive cartilage has been removed during the operative procedure, replacing a portion of the excised cartilage as an onlay graft is the best option. If revision surgery is required, autogenous cartilage can be used to repair larger defects. Small defects may be corrected with alloplastic materials if they can be placed in a surgically sterile pocket. Leaving an adequate strut of cartilaginous septum is important to prevent the postoperative collapse of the nasal vault. If submucous resection of the cartilaginous septum is necessary, the surgeon must also allow for dorsal hump resection. An adequate L-shaped strut of cartilage, usually at least 1 cm, must remain for nasal support after both procedures.

Underreduction of the cartilaginous vault may produce a persistent dorsal hump or pollybeak

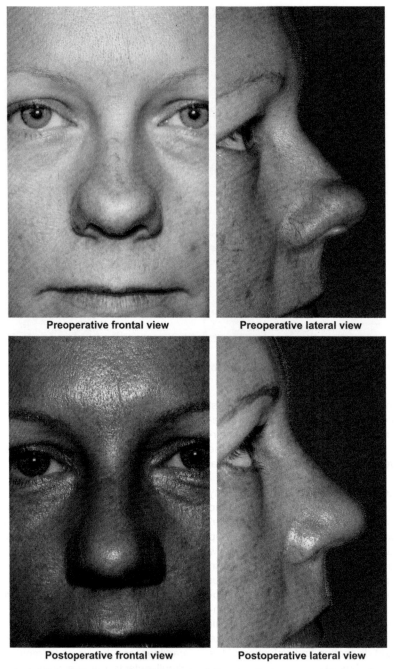

Preoperative frontal view   **Preoperative lateral view**

Postoperative frontal view   **Postoperative lateral view**

Fig. 5. An interrupted strip technique was used for maximal tip retrodisplacement. The lateral crura were divided, a portion was excised, and then it was reconstituted.

deformity.[13] Again, careful evaluation of the nasal tip as it relates to the cartilaginous and bony dorsum at original surgery can minimize these problems. Occasionally, pollybeak deformities may develop over time if the tip becomes more ptotic postoperatively. Maintaining adequate tip support mechanisms during the surgical procedure to prevent postoperative loss of tip projection. Typically,

the nasal tip will settle slightly postoperatively so the surgeon must ensure adequate cartilaginous hump removal during the initial procedure (**Fig. 6**). The pollybeak deformity may also be relative to overresection of the bony dorsum. Treatment of the pollybeak deformity depends on the actual cause. If the pollybeak deformity is a result of inadequate cartilaginous hump removal, then

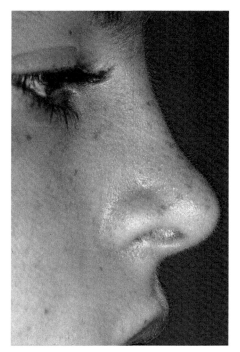

Fig. 6. A slight pollybeak remains as a result of inadequate reduction of the dorsal cartilage.

additional hump resection may be necessary. If the pollybeak deformity is a result of tip ptosis the insertion of a columellar strut may be beneficial. If the bony hump was overresected, then augmentation to the bony dorsum may be necessary. Finally, occasionally the pollybeak deformity may be a result of excessive scar formation. If the dead space of the supratip area is not stabilized by proper splinting then postoperative fluid accumulation may occur, resulting in excessive fibrosis and scarring. The subcutaneous injection of triamcinolone may be helpful in these cases.

Cartilaginous vault abnormalities may also arise from the upper lateral cartilages. If there is inadequate support of the upper lateral cartilages after dorsal hump removal, they may collapse and produce an inverted V deformity.[14] The nasal mucoperichondrium can provide significant support to the upper lateral cartilages and may help decrease the risk for collapse of the upper lateral cartilages after hump excision. It is also possible to produce abnormalities of the upper lateral cartilages by dislocating them from the undersurface of the nasal bones. It is important to remember the relationship of the caudal nasal bones and the underlying upper lateral cartilages. Excessive use of a bony rasp can accidentally avulse and disarticulate the cartilage. This will produce a visual step-off depression requiring camouflage.

The Bony Vault

Underreduction of the bony vault results in a continued dorsal hump deformity postoperatively. Typically a stronger dorsal profile is preferable to an overreduced nasal profile. If additional surgery is required, correcting the underreduction is much easier than repairing an overreduction. Depending on the amount of additional reduction required, simple rasping of the dorsal hump may be sufficient to lower the hump to its desired position. If a more extensive removal is required, then lateral osteotomies may be required to properly narrow the nose and prevent an open roof deformity.

Overreduction of the bony dorsum will result in a saddle deformity (**Fig. 7**). The overreduction may also involve the cartilaginous portion of the nasal dorsum. Surgical correction requires onlay grafting with autogenous cartilage. Preparing a precise pocket in the nasal dorsum when correcting these deformities is important. An overly large pocket will invite shifting and displacement of the graft material. The pocket should be developed to allow for the thickest possible soft tissue covering over the graft. This procedure will lessen the likelihood of smaller irregularities being visible through the dorsal skin.

Asymmetrical abnormalities of the bony vault may also be present. Uneven osteotomies, asymmetrical hump removal, rocker deformities, and

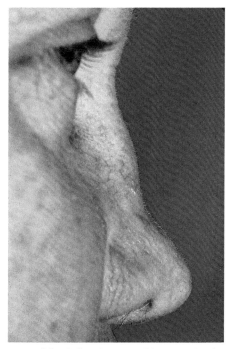

Fig. 7. A saddle deformity caused by excessive loss of the bony and cartilaginous dorsum.

persistent bony ridges may become apparent postoperatively. If, during the original surgery, the bony hump is removed with an osteotome, it should be inspected to ensure an even amount of bone removal. Rocker deformities may occur if the lateral osteotomies are taken too high into the thick frontal bone. When the bone is then infractured, it may rock at the superior fracture site. As the surgeon digitally displaces the fractured bone medially, the superior portion will actually rock laterally. This can be corrected with a small osteotome from a percutaneous approach. The open roof deformity results from the failure to close the space between the lateral nasal bones after hump removal. A cross-section of the nose will appear as a trapezoid instead of the more natural triangular configuration. Correction of this deformity requires closing the space between the lateral nasal bones. If the nasal dorsum has been overreduced in addition to the open roof deformity, an autogenous graft might also be necessary. If minimal hump removal has occurred, then medial osteotomies may also be needed to close the open roof deformity.

Persistent nasal deviations may remain postoperatively in patients. Correction of the deviated nose presents a difficult challenge. Usually an aesthetic concern is present in addition to a functional problem. Abnormalities in the nasal septum are usually a major component of the deviation and must be adequately addressed.[15] The nasal bone will usually require mobilization through asymmetric osteotomies.

Abnormalities of the soft tissue envelope may also occur. Rhinoplasty should be performed in the proper tissue planes. Performing dissection in too superficial a plane can damage the vascular supply to the overlying skin of the nose. It also produces a bloodier surgical field, which is more difficult to operate in. If the soft tissue envelope is damaged it is impossible to fully repair, and if the scar retraction is severe it can lead to a complication known as the *crucified tip*. Loss of vestibular skin and heavy scarring of the cutaneous tissue may occur, producing an amorphous tip with severe contraction and retraction. Repair of this deformity can be extremely difficult and may require multiple full-thickness grafts to replace missing tissue.[16] The residual blood supply is usually compromised and healing will be prolonged and less predictable than normal.

Complications in cosmetic surgery can be particularly distressing to patients. Generally, healthy patients have decided to undergo a surgical treatment so that an esthetic improvement might occur. Complications can adversely affect the surgical outcome, and typically those that arise from overly aggressive surgery are more difficult to treat than those caused by too conservative a procedure.

Because rhinoplasty involves the healing dynamics of different tissue types, an element of unpredictability will always be present. Surgeons are responsible for limiting this unpredictability as much as possible, and can develop a graduated systematic approach through carefully evaluating patients preoperatively. In cosmetic surgery the ultimate goal is to make the patient happy, which may be accomplished by either producing the results the patient desires or educating them as to why these results are not possible.

Each rhinoplasty will have its own set of goals. Surgeons must decide whether tip projection is to be reduced, maintained, or enhanced, and whether the tip volume, rotation, or symmetry should be altered. Similar goals must be established for the treatment of the cartilaginous and bony dorsum, and then surgeons must decide which incisions to use. These incisions must provide adequate access to allow predictable modification of the nasal structures. Typically, years of experience are required to thoroughly understand and master refinement of the nasal tip. The final result is not visualized for many months or years after the procedure. Through long-term follow-up and careful patient examination, surgeons will gain a better understanding of the consequences of surgical manipulation. Using standardized pre- and postsurgical photographs along with objective analysis of the results will ultimately speed this process.

REFERENCES

1. Rees TD. Postoperative considerations and complications. In: Rees TD, editor. Aesthetic plastic surgery. Philadelphia: Saunders; 1980. p. 337.
2. Becker DG. Complications in rhinoplasty. In: Papel I, editor. Facial plastic and reconstructive surgery. 2nd edition. New York: Thieme; 2002.
3. Webster RC. Revisional rhinoplasty. Otolaryngol Clin North Am 1975;8(3):753–82.
4. Busca GP, Amasio ME, Satoris A. Complications of rhinoplasty. Acta Otorhinolaryngol Ital 1990;10(31): 1–37.
5. Holt GR, Garner ET, McLarey D. Postoperative sequelae and complications of rhinoplasty. Otolaryngol Clin North Am 1987;20(4):853–76.
6. Tardy ME, Denneny JC. Micro-osteotomes in rhinoplasty. Facial Plast Surg 1984;1(2):137–45.
7. Becker DG, Becker SS. Reducing complications in rhinoplasty. Otolaryngol Clin North Am 2006;39(3): 475–92.

8. Thomas JR, Tardy ME. Complications of rhinoplasty. Ear Nose Throat J 1986;65:19–34.

9. Toriumi DM, Josen J, Weinberger MS, et al. Use of alar batten grafts for correction of nasal valve collapse. Arch Otolaryngol Head Neck Surg 1997; 123:802–8.

10. Tardy ME, Toriumi DM. Alar retraction: composite graft correction. Facial Plast Surg 1989;6:101–7.

11. Stucker FJ, Bryarly RC, Shockley WW. The failed rhinoplasty. Current therapy in otolaryngology head and neck surgery 1984–1985. Philadelphia: Decker; 1984. p. 129–34.

12. Hewell TS, Tardy ME. Nasal tip refinement. Facial Plast Surg 1984;2:87–124.

13. Kamer FM, McQuown SA. Revision rhinoplasty. Analysis and treatment. Arch Otolaryngol Head Neck Surg 1988;114:257–66.

14. Toriumi DM. Management of the middle nasal vault. Oper Tech Plast Recontr Surg 1995;2:16–30.

15. Stucker FJ. Management of the scoliotic nose. Laryngoscope 1982;92(2):128–34.

16. Tardy ME, Cheng EY, Jenstrom V. Misadventures in nasal tip surgery. Otolaryngol Clin North Am 1987; 20(4):797–823.

Complications of Facial Implants

L. Angelo Cuzalina, MD, DDS*, Matthew R. Hlavacek, MD, DDS

KEYWORDS

- Alloplast • Malar implant • Mandibular implant
- Facial implant • Complications

Volume replacement and contour augmentation of the face have been pillars of facial surgery for cosmetic, as well as traumatic, congenital, and extirpative defect correction. The endpoint goal of such treatment must be an aesthetic result. As such, the public's preference for facial beauty has evolved over time. This change has been demonstrated by the desire for different cosmetic procedures by the public. The art and science of facial cosmetic and reconstructive surgery have evolved to meet this need. This evolution is reflected in the drive to create less invasive surgical options for facial augmentation, including the development of alloplastic materials.

According to the American Society of Plastic Surgeons member survey, in 1990 the most commonly augmented facial sites where implants were used were the nasal dorsum, chin and malar eminence, in descending order. The 2005 American Academy of Cosmetic Surgery procedural census showed that malar implants were more commonly being performed than genial implants.

Autologous tissues should be the gold standard against which alloplastic implantation for facial augmentation should be judged. Drawbacks of autogenous grafting include: donor site morbidity, limited availability, limited moldability, and unpredictable resorption.[1] Alloplastic materials, however, have their own set of potential problems. For an alloplastic implant to be successfully placed, the implant must be made out of a material that has low enough bioactivity or toxicity that the body will not reject it. It must be stable and strong enough to withstand the physiologic milieu of changes that occur in the body. It must be used and placed appropriately by the surgeon and there must be a favorable recipient site with adequate healing potential by the patient.[2] Shortcomings in any of these conditions can lead to complications. An understanding of these qualities is needed to adequately prevent complications or to treat them when they occur.

ALLOPLASTIC AUGMENTATION MATERIALS

The surgeon must be able to make an informed decision regarding the selection of a synthetic implant based on chemical composition, physical structure, and planned site for application. Characteristics of an ideal implant include: biocompatibility, chemical inertness, lack of elicitation of foreign body or hypersensitivity reaction, noncarcinogenic, and easily shaped.[3] The ideal implant integrates into the surrounding hard and soft tissues. Fulfilling these goals will minimize complications.

The biocompatibility of the material is central to its suitability for implantation. If a material is not accepted by the native tissues, adverse reaction or rejection may ensue. In even the best results with alloplastic implants, a mild foreign body reaction occurs which results in fibrous encapsulation and/or biointegration. Successful implantation is determined by the implant's chemical composition, surface characteristics at both the macroscopic and microscopic levels, mechanical properties, and biostability (**Fig. 1**).

The intrinsic inertness of the material is a major factor affecting the severity of the inflammatory response. The most inert materials are those composed of elements nearest calcium and carbon on the periodic table because these elements compose the greatest nonwater part of the human body.[4] Elemental composition of the implant may be one of the most important factors in determining the host response; implants made of increasingly reactive elements are toxic and rejected.

Tulsa Surgical Arts, 7322 E. 91st Street, Tulsa, OK 74133, USA
* Corresponding author.
E-mail address: angelo@tulsasurgicalarts.com (L.A. Cuzalina).

Oral Maxillofacial Surg Clin N Am 21 (2009) 91–104
doi:10.1016/j.coms.2008.10.009
1042-3699/08/$ – see front matter © 2009 Elsevier Inc. All rights reserved.

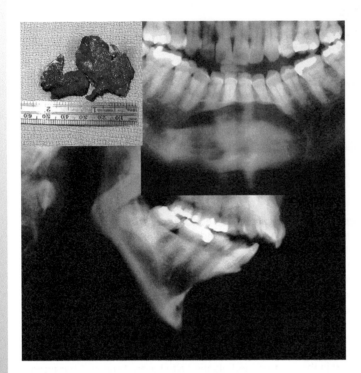

Fig. 1. A severe inflammatory response with massive bone resorbtion is shown when an older form of mesh material placed in this patient longer than a decade before removal of the implant material. The large defect eroded into the adjacent teeth. Mesh and other porous implant materials are usually difficult to surgically remove because of tissue in growth and associated peri-implant fibrosis.

On a macroscopic level, porous implants like polytetrafluoroethylene (PTFE), high molecular weight polyethylene (HMWPE) and meshes have the advantage of fibrous tissue in growth and fixation. Smooth implants like silicone and polymethylmethacrylate (PMMA) are nonporous and become encapsulated. Encapsulation of smooth implants and their predisposition to movement are directly or indirectly responsible for the majority of their late complications. However, the nonporous implants have a distinct advantage related to infection because bacteria is much less likely to penetrate the nonporous implant compared with porous implants.

On a microscopic level, pore size of the material is significant in nonsmooth implants. Bacteria are excluded from porous materials with a pore size less than 1 micrometer. Additionally, a pore size of over 50 micrometers is required for migration of macrophages into the material. Thus, materials with pore sizes of 1–50 micrometers are at an increased risk for infection. Pore sizes greater than 100 micrometers facilitate soft tissue in growth and fixation. This feature is also important for delivering immune mediators to prevent and resolve infections.

The surface irregularity of the implant may also impart an energy that can increase the adsorption of cells and proteins including bacteria and immunoresponsive cells. This is evidenced by the fact that highly surface–reactive implants may elicit a host tissue response characterized by a higher proportion of macrophage activity, inflammatory response, wound breakdown and potential extrusion.[5]

PROBLEMS RELATED TO SPECIFIC ANATOMIC SITES
Malar Implants

Strong cheekbones give the face a fresh and youthful look that contributes to facial harmony. Hypoplastic cheekbones or atrophic submalar regions contribute to an aged appearance on even relatively young individuals. The addition of malar, submalar or combination cheek implants can do wonders in rejuvenating the look of an ideal patient. However, because humans have two cheeks rather than one, complications related to cheek implants tend to be much higher than that for isolated chin implants. Minor asymmetry is the most common problem.

According to the 1990 ASPRS survey, the following complications were reported for malar implants in order of decreasing frequency: patient/doctor dissatisfaction, asymmetry, malposition, hematoma/seroma/infection, extrusion, and nerve dysfunction.

In Wilkinsons[5] retrospective evaluation of postoperative complications in 35 of his patients who underwent malar implants, he felt that incorrect choice of the point of prominence was at fault for his most common problem of error in placement.

Malar and submalar implants can be placed through intra-oral, subciliary, transconjunctival, or rhytidectomy approaches. The intra-oral approach obviously offers the advantage of a hidden scar. The drawbacks include: 1) the implant is contaminated with saliva; and, 2) the posterior aspect of the dissection can be blind and more difficult. According to Terino, complications from an intra-oral approach should occur in less than 0.5% of cases He feels that the intra-oral approach creates incisional weakness inferiorly in the muscle floor, which increases the chance of rotational asymmetries and medial inferior descent of the implant without fixation.[6] With approaches other than transoral, more flexible materials should be considered. This is primarily due to limited dissection and difficulty with access and fixation. The benefits of malar implant placement through a subciliary incision are that: it allows accurate visualization of the implant placement; it minimizes contamination; and it provides a sturdy inferior cheek shell on which the implant can rest. Periorbital routes can be associated with a higher rate of epiphora, ectropion, infraorbital nerve neuropraxia, and subconjunctival bruising.[7] Also, the cheek implant is more likely to "ride up" with this route of insertion (**Fig. 2**). The rhytidectomy approach offers advantages of sterile entry wound and reasonable opportunity for accurate placement, but it may be difficult gaining access posteriorly to the temporal dissection of the zygomatic arch, thus increasing buckling of the implant. Also, this approach is not really an option unless a facelift is also being performed. Disadvantages of facial versus oral access are: the facial access risks injury to the facial and infraorbital nerves in the case of malar implants; potentially less than ideal exposure; and external scars.[8]

Mandibular

Microgenia conveys weakness and femininity where as strong chins convey power,

determination, and masculinity. Chin implants are used to treat a recessive chin, recessive procumbent lower lip, exaggerated labiomental fold and prejowel sulcus, and diminished lower facial height.

According to the 1990 ASPRS Survey, the frequency of complications with chin implants in descending order are: asymmetry, malposition, hematoma/seroma/infection, mobility, extrusion, and nerve dysfunction. The sensory innervation was affected to a greater extent than motor. Additional potential complications include: displacement, bone resorption, soft tissue ptosis or distortion of the overlying soft tissue, and patient dislike. The overall complication rate as per a retrospective study by Gross and colleagues[9] involving 264 mersilene chin augmentations using both intra and extraoral approaches was 2.3%.

Chin implants can be placed via intra-oral or extra-oral approach. Obvious benefit to the intra-oral approach is avoidance of an extra-oral scar; however, the mentalis undergoes instrumentation and the implant is contaminated with saliva. In a study done by Scaccia and colleagues[10] involving 11,095 mentoplasty procedures, the researchers found that the infection rate was slightly higher with the intra-oral approach, but the malposition rate was lower. They thought that this was due to superior exposure allowing more precise placement of the implant. The larger dissection for the intra-oral route can result in more postoperative pain and swelling compared with an extraoral, submental incision. Failure to reapproximate the mentalis adequately can lead to chin ptosis and what is otherwise known as a "witches chin deformity" (**Fig. 3**) Proponents of the external access think that the scar is well camouflaged; there is decreased trauma to the mentalis; and there is minimization of superior dissection and, thus, potential for migration.[11] This approach is definitely indicated if a preexisting submental scar is present or if submental liposuction is to be performed at the same time. In a rather extensive review of the

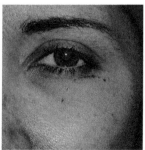
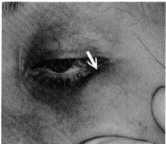
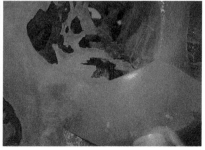

Fig. 2. The left cheek implant seen here can be easily palpated and is objectionable to the patient when in close proximity to the orbital rim. Malar or tear trough implants placed via a subcilliary or transconjuctival approach are more likely to "ride up" along the rim than implants placed via the transoral route.

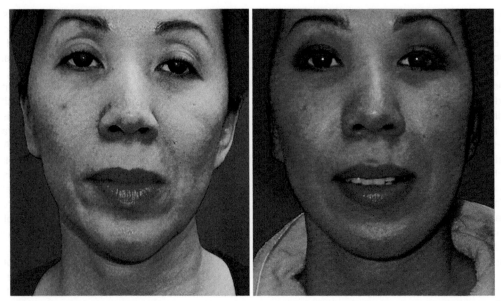

Fig. 3. A "witches chin" deformity with narrowing at the pre-jowl sulcus bilaterally seen here on the left was likely a result from transection of the mentalis muscle along with placement of an old "button" style chin implant. Correction of the deformity shown on the right was performed by removal of the button style implant and replacement using a proper fitting "anatomic" style chin implant with screw fixation.

literature, Rubin and Yarmechuck discovered that a unique feature of chin implant complications was that they have the potential to occur late in the postoperative period, up to almost 50 years after insertion.[12] Some surgeons feel that dental and periodontal health are the culprits for these late infections and that this must be screened for before placement.[13]

The mandibular angle gives definition to the face and separates the posterior face from the neck. Osteotomies to increase posterior facial or ramus height are unstable and access is difficult; as

a result, alloplastic augmentation gets much more consideration. Mandibular angle implants can be used to flatten or decrease a steep mandibular plane angle, especially when used in concert with genial augmentation (**Fig. 4**). In Yarmechuck's report of 11 patients who underwent porous polyethylene angle implants placed transorally, there was no infection, no exposure, and no nerve deficit for patients with a follow-up average of two years. One patient required another operation to correct poor transition at the inferior boarder.[14] Mandibular angle implants are some

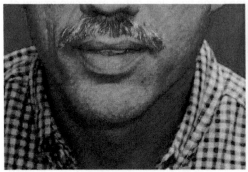
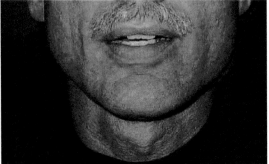

Fig. 4. In general, mandibular angle and cheek implants are the most likely of all facial implants to result in postoperative asymmetry. Occasionally implants can improve symmetry issues. Mandibular angle implants and a chin implant were used here to add facial volume and improve preoperative asymmetry that existed before any implant placement as seen on the left.

of most difficult implants to position because of the location and because they are inherently more prone to mild asymmetries.

Nasal

Dorsal nasal implants are used in revision rhinoplasty and also primary augmentation in African American and Asian patients.[15] Nasal augmentation has similar issues to augmentation of other areas of the face. The most important determinant of the long-term success of an alloplastic dorsal nasal implant is the amount of skin covering it. The thicker, more vascularized skin has less risk for implant visibility and extrusion.

The overall incidence of complications after augmentation rhinoplasty with silicone implants can be as high as 36%.[16] This includes discoloration, dislocation, extrusion, capsular contracture, and infection (**Fig. 5**). Early complications are primarily due to implant size or placement position; in contrast, late complications are primarily due to tissue reaction. In a retrospective study by Deva and colleagues[17] 422 patients underwent silastic nasal augmentation. 9.7% percent developed postoperative complications that required implant removal. The most common reason for removal was displacement or overprominence.

Some authors believe that malposition is the most common complication after silicone nasal dorsal augmentation. This can be a result of capsular contracture, which has a higher incidence when implants are placed in the soft tissue versus a subperiosteal or subperichondrial plane. As mentioned previously, the most likely reason for problems is related to inadequate soft tissue coverage.

COMPLICATIONS
Improper Selection or Placement

Generally speaking, improper placement of the implant is the most common complication followed by improper implant selection. These complications can include selecting to place an implant in a patient who is not necessarily a good candidate (**Fig. 6**). Patients are as dissatisfied with improper size, shape, or contour as they are with asymmetry. The implant should be slightly smaller than the desired increase in fullness to take the contribution of the soft tissue into account. Appropriate implant selection is also important because, for example, selecting too large an implant will lead to excessive soft tissue tension, which could lead to ischemia, necrosis, or extrusion.

Placement of malar implants in too lateral a position can cause the eyes to look too close together. Placing the implants too medial and inferior will give a look of "chipmunk cheeks." In a study by Metzinger and colleagues[18] involving 118 implants, one silastic malar implant was placed in the wrong orientation and one patient requested a larger size. He owed his low incidence of complications in this respect to minimal dissection, frequent intraoperative evaluation, and suture fixation. In a retrospective study of 11,095 mentoplasty procedures, the most common complication was malposition with the subperiosteal approach slightly lower than supraperiosteal.

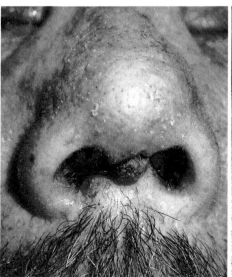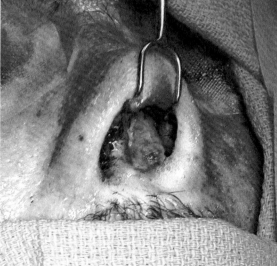

Fig. 5. Extruded silicone nasal implant.

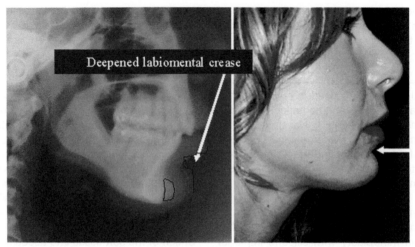

Fig. 6. A chin implant will likely worsen an already deep labiomental groove. Patients with severe mandibular hypoplasia and a deep bite may be inappropriate candidates for chin implant camouflage if the depth of labiomental crease is severe.

This problem is understandable considering the mobility provided by an extra layer of soft tissue.

Neuropraxia

According to the ASPRS Survey in 1990, 8% of surgeons reported nerve complications in patients following malar augmentation versus 10% with genial augmentation. The malar neuropraxias had a slightly higher ratio of motor nerve injuries than sensory. Neuropraxia can be incurred from impingement by the implant because a size selection that is too large, migration, improper placement, a traction injury, a thermal injury, or a direct traumatic injury from dissection. Most patients regain sensation and function within three weeks. Anesthesia postimplant placement probably indicates the implant is resting on the nerve.

Dissection for Malar implants involves elevating tissue around the infraorbital nerve, which supplies sensation to the midface from the lower lid to the upper lip. Dissection to visualize this nerve is usually not required unless an orbital rim or tear trough implant is being placed. Thus, for the more commonly used malar, submalar, or combo implants, it is rare for patients to develop sensation change in the cheek due to neuropraxia of the infraorbital nerve. Dissection for malar implants can also involve instrumentation around the facial nerve branches. Weakness of the zygomaticus, orbicularis oculi, or the frontalis muscles can be induced by disturbance of the temporofrontal branch of the facial nerve while dissecting posteriorly over the middle third of the zygomatic arch. Also, not staying subperiosteal in this area predisposes to misadventerous dissection into the parotid and facial nerve branches and/or facial musculature.

During dissection of the chin for genial alloplast placement, it is important to avoid the mental nerve, which is approximately underneath the area of the premolars intraorally. It fans superior and posterior from its foramen to innervate the lower lip and chin area. The sheath is quite durable and a traction injury is much more likely than an avulsion. Mental nerve injuries are exceedingly rare as evidenced by a review of complications associated with 11,095 mentoplasty cases where no single incidence of neuropraxia was reported. The marginal mandibular branch of the facial nerve, which supplies muscles of the lower lip and chin, is above the periosteum over the inferior boarder of the mandible and is difficult to injure unless there is a sever traction injury or perforation of the periosteum. Subperiosteal dissection along the inferior mandibular boarder, in addition to screw placement that avoids tooth roots and the path of the inferior alveolar nerve, will prevent concomitant related sensation changes.

Edema and Ecchymosis

Typically the majority of postoperative edema and ecchymosis resolves in two weeks, but edema can persist for 6 months and even up to a year.[19] In a study on malar implants, Metzinger reported persistent edema, which took up to 6 months to resolve. Implant fixation is important because excessive continuing movement can cause tissue injury, chronic inflammation, and suboptimal soft tissue acceptance with prolonged edema (**Fig. 7**). This could also be due to a nonspecific

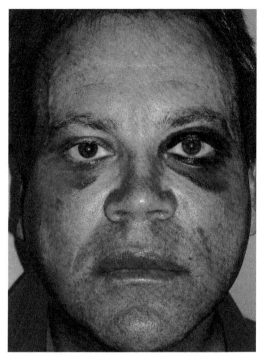

Fig. 7. Unexpected ecchymosis following cheek implant placement.

immune reaction to the implant material. Persistent swelling is more commonly associated with mandibular than malar implants.

Hematoma and Seroma

Abnormal fluid collection can be the result of inadequate hemostasis, overdissection, traumatic handling of the tissues, dead space around or underneath the implant, elevated blood pressure from any number of factors including pain, secondary trauma to the operative site, and secondary procedures. Hematomas and seromas encourage the growth of bacterial contamination potentiating cellulitis and subsequent fullminant infection (**Fig. 8**). Blood or seromatous fluid collection can also imitate postoperative asymmetries, thereby confusing this issue. They can result in excessive fibrosis producing soft tissue defects. In the worst-case scenario, they can cause a pressure effect on the overlaying soft tissue and skin, compromising blood flow and resulting in necrosis.

Smaller hematomas (<5 cc) resolve without treatment in 10–14 days. Large hematomas need to be recognized and evacuated with the implant removed as necessary. Seromas usually present around 2 weeks after surgery. Presence of

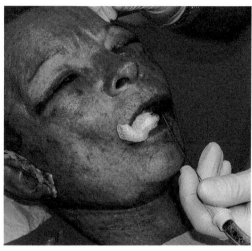

Fig. 8. Immediate recognition and surgical evacuation of a hematoma around facial implants is critical to prevent future problems. Intraoral suction assisted evacuation of a hematoma around the left cheek implant is shown the day after surgery.

liquefied hematomas or seromas 2–4 weeks postoperatively may be drained percutaneously.

Hematomas and seromas are best prevented with control of blood pressure during the procedure with general anesthesia and adequate local anesthesia, postoperatively with antihypertensive prophylaxis, and gentle handling of the tissues, maintaining a subperiosteal plane, and consideration for a drain in secondary procedures. Fixation also eliminates the gaps between the implant and the skeleton that could result in unplanned increases in augmentation and the creation of dead space for hematoma or seroma formation.[20]

Infection

There are many different factors that determine whether an infection will be propagated after an implant is contaminated. Some of these factors include the bacterial load of contamination, host factors such as immune function, the method of contamination and age of the implant, and the perioperative prophylactic interventions by the surgeon to prevent infection. Implants can be contaminated by hematogenous, contiguous spread, or direct inoculation.

Rubin and Yarmechuck's extensive review of available literature found an infection rate of 3.8% with silastic implants, 0.9% for porous polyethylene, and 2.2% for ePTFE for mixed facial sites, for an overall infection rate of 3%. The average infection rate for chin implants was 1.4%. They found that silicone chin implants have an infection rate of 0.7% with mesh and proplast demonstrating higher rates and porous polyethylene lower. The overall infection rate for malar implants was 2.4%, including a rate of 1.2% for silicone. The overall infection rate for nasal implants was 2.4%. This rate was lowest for silicone and highest for polyethylene and mesh.

Implants decrease the amount of bacterial innoculum required to produce an infection. Foreign bodies have been shown to reduce the number of bacteria required to produce an infection by 10^4 to 10^6 power.[21] Zimerli found that decreased overall bactericidal activity, including opsonization, bacterial ingestion, and intracellular killing of bacteria in neutrophils exposed to a foreign body.[22]

Numerous biomaterial characteristics influence the potential for implant contamination and subsequent infection. These include chemical composition, surface roughness, surface configuration, and hydrobobicity. Hydropillic materials are more resistant to adhesion than hydrophobic materials. Scalfani and colleagues studied the infection susceptibility of implants with different pore sizes. They found that the PTFE with an average pore size of 22 microns became infected at lower innoculum counts and sooner than polyethylene with a pore size of 150 microns. Biomaterial surface configuration may confer resistance to infection depending upon when the implant is infected. Most infections in the early postoperative time period are more likely to occur with porous implants because of increased surface area, irregularity, and surface energy, which facilitates glycolax formation and bacterial adherence. Late infections are less likely to occur with porous implants because of incorporation of host tissue and improved immune response. Coverage with and ingrowth of host tissue also reduces the space available for bacterial implantation and makes a significant immune system contribution.

Infections that occur years after surgery are most probably caused by hematogenous spread or direct violation of the implant capsule with bacterial seeding like an injection needle. Late infection associated with malar implants have been associated with dental injections as reported by Cohen and Kawamoto.[23] In Wilkinson's retrospective review of 35 malar implant patients, he had two patients who developed late infection at 8 months and 2 years, respectively, which he thought were associated with old hematoma and subsequently cultured Staphylococcus aureaus. One implant had to be removed and the other patient responded to oral antibiotics.[5]

Some authors hypothesize that exposure to saliva confers enough risk for development of infection that the intra-oral route should be avoided. In a study by Deva and colleagues, 422 patients had silastic nasal augmentation consisting of primarily columellar struts using an intraoral approach without prophylactic antibiotics. No patients developed postoperative infections. Karras and Wolford[24] reported on 18 patients who had hard tissue replacement polymer (HTR) chin implants placed through the mouth with perioperative and postoperative antibiotics and reported no incidence of infection. These studies support the idea that patients with an intact immune system and healthy wound bed do not need additional antibiotics.

One would think that if transoral placement predisposes to contamination and infection, those procedures where incisions were made in the lower sulcus of the lip or cheek would expose the implant to the most salivary percolation and thus have the highest infection rates (**Fig. 9**). As demonstrated by Yarmechuck, this is not the case. In his series of 11 mandibular angle implants placed through the mouth, he had no postoperative infections. He attributed this to making the incision slightly out of the bottom of the sulcus and also to his two-layered watertight closure.

After a purulent infection is established, the biofilm is resistant to antibiotics; drainage and removal are typically necessary. S. aureus is the main pathogen and is usually susceptible to penicillin or cephalosporin. A better chance of eradicating the infection with antibiotics and drainage is possible with nonporous implants. Terino believes that silastic implants can survive gross infection and inflammation where as porous

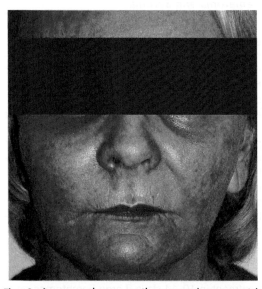

Fig. 9. As seen here, erythema and asymmetric changes are early signs of this infected right cheek implant. High suspicion is required for early diagnosis and treatment.

implants such as ePTFE and HWMPE cannot and must be removed. This author has seen similar results with nonporous silicone implants, which often can be salvaged from infection if caught early and if the implant has good fixation to avoid mobility in an infected pocket. Scalfani reports that, with more fibrous tissue in growth and maturation, a later onset infection associated with a porous implant may deserve more consideration for conservative treatment before removal.

If salvage is selected in the setting of a purulent infection, the implant should be removed and scrubbed and/or sterilized to remove the biofilm. In addition, debridement and copious irrigation of the implant pocket and, finally, a prolonged postoperative antibiotic course are advocated. If rapid improvement does not occur and the implant needs to be removed, it should not be replaced for 6–8 weeks to allow for resolution of the infection and inflammation.[25] Expect difficulty when removing porous implants because of the fibrous tissue in growth.

Migration and Contour Changes

In Rubin and Yarmechuck's review of the literature, they found an overall displacement rate of 2.3% for various types of alloplasts, which were used primarily for malar and chin augmentation; 2% for silicone. They hypothesized that this was highly influenced by implant shape and method of fixation. Displacement is roughly equal when comparing genial augmentation to malar. In a study by Metzinger and colleagues involving 118 silastic malar implants, four underwent displacement, two requiring revision (**Fig. 10**). The rate of displacement may be higher for nasal implants. In the study by Deva and colleagues reviewing the placement

of 422 silastic nasal implants which were primarily columellar struts, displacement was the cause of 4% of prosthesis removals, occurring primarily in the first month after placement.

Although some practitioners have advocated retention without fixation in the past and have relied on implant design and soft tissue ledges and pockets, fixation is integral to preventing migration. Migration is usually the result of overdissection, selection of the wrong-sized implant, and lack of fixation—for example, implants that are too small or placed in an overdissected pocket. Supraperiosteal placement can also predispose the implant to mobility especially without adequate fixation (**Fig. 11**).

Anatomic implants have decreased the potential for migration, rotation, and displacement because of their expansion in size to volumetrically match the surface area of the zones to be augmented. Also, as previously mentioned, subperiosteal placement and screw or suture fixation help to prevent migration.

Delayed contour changes have been reported in association with silastic augmentation. This is thought to be associated with capsular contracture around the implant in addition to calcification of the capsule itself. In the study by Jung where 221 silastic nasal implants were removed during revision rhinoplasty from 1–25 years postopeatively, some form of calcification was found in the capsule or on the implant itself, causing increased firmness of the implant or distortion of nasal form.

Extrusion

Factors which are critical to preventing extrusion include adequate soft tissue bulk with quality

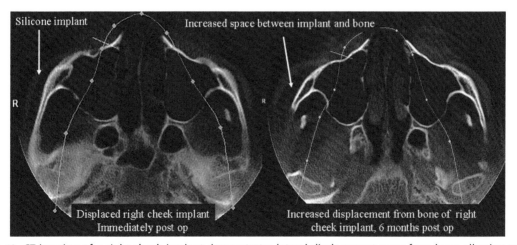

Fig. 10. CT imaging of a right cheek implant demonstrates lateral displacement away from bone allowing soft tissue in growth and facial asymmetry.

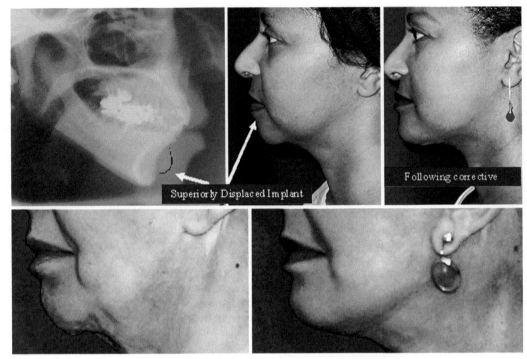

Fig. 11. The top figure demonstrates a superiorly displaced chin implant corrected by repositioning and placement of a larger anatomic implant with screw fixation. The lower figure shows an inferiorly displaced chin implant beneath the jaw requiring removal and replacement using screw fixation.

tissue for cover and insertion in the correct plane without tension. Decreased tissue perfusion decreases the potential for successful wound healing. Factors such as prior surgery and history of radiation will decrease the local vascular supply and result in fibrosis and stiffening of the tissues. Highly scarred and thinned tissues tend to atrophy over time and are at a higher risk for postoperative infection, exposure, and extrusion.[26]

Excessive tension is usually the result of using too large an implant for too small a dissection. In addition to tensionless closure, subperiosteal placement helps to prevent exposure. For example, placement of chin implants supraperiosteally or without fixation allows for micromovement due to activation of the mentalis. This will ultimately lead to erosion into the body of the mandible and/or chronic infection with extrusion. Skin and dermis alone are rarely adequate for implant cover and implants usually need to be buried under a layer of subcutaneous fat or muscle.

Rubin and Yarmechuck found that the overall extrusion rate was 5.2%, highest for silicone implants at 22.7% and lowest for more compliant materials like mesh. The restriction of the soft tissue of the nose places this anatomic site at the highest risk for extrusion. In the study by Deva and colleagues reviewing the placement of 422 silastic nasal implants that were primarily columellar struts, he theorized that the primary reason for extrusion was overaugmentation.

Some biomaterials can be treated symptomatically if exposure occurs without the need for removal. Frodel and Lee report secondary healing over polyethylene implant exposure and believe that if there is adequate vascularity, the implant will do well.[27] Other authors report intra-oral exposure of silastic implants that go on to cover secondarily with local wound care. Typically, however, if extrusion occurs, the implant must be removed and the site allowed to heal for multiple weeks before replacement.

Palpability

Even the most perfect augmentation will be a failure if the patient can feel the implant and does not like it. This can be the result of improper size selection or contour, improper positioning, improperly placed fixation, or capsular contracture. Patient factors such as a thin amount of overlying tissue also predispose to palpability. In malar augmentation, Whitaker recommends limiting the thickness of the implant to no greater then 4–5 mm and tapering the ends thinly to avoid palpability. Although this is obviously not applicable to all alloplastic facial augmentation situations, the underlying principle is that less may be best.[28]

It is important to make sure the implants are intimately adapted before fixation. With anatomic chin implants, the thinner posterolateral limb can rotate under the mandibular boarder if it is over dissected or it can buckle if not properly inserted, becoming palpable and creating an abnormal external contour. Yarmechuck advocates final contouring of the implant after fixation.

Lip dysfunction

Altered lip function is primarily associated with malar implants. This problem occurs because dissection can interfere with the muscles responsible for smiling mimetics, more so than for mandibular augmentation. Other factors could include edema, interposition of a solid implant which stretches the muscles of the midface, or interference with the facial nerve during dissection over the zygomatic arch. Whitaker noted a sense of reduced lip mobility for 6–8 weeks in his retrospective study of 176 malar implants placed by the intra-oral route. He used a short (1.5 cm) horizontal vestibular incision with a more generous dissection. In all patients except one, lip mimetics returned to normal.

As mentioned previously, postoperative edema can also be a significant factor and becomes maximal at 72 hours. The edema can cause dysfunction in the muscles of the upper lip resembling facial nerve dysfunction. The edema usually subsides with in a few days. When dysfunction is due to muscle displacement, it usually takes 1–3 months for the muscles to reattach and the capsule to become soft and distensible.

In malar augmentation, upper lip weakness can be minimized by a small, vertical mucosal incision and dissection parallel to and in between the zygomaticus major and minor, as well as by careful and limited subperiosteal dissection particularly along the posterior zygomatic arch.

Bone resorption

Bone erosion under alloplastic implants may have occurred to a significant extent with early implants (**Fig. 12**). Robinson first reported bone resorption under silastic and acrylic chin implants in 12 of 14 patients at up to 5 mm in 48 months.[29] These early reports were more commonly associated with chin button style or centrally placed implants. The bone resorption was often attributed to foreign body giant cell reaction between the implant and the bone or to pressure from the mentalis muscle against the implant. Other factors that were considered were improper implant positioning, pressure due to an oversized implant, subperiosteal placement and hardness of the implant. Significant resorption poses not only an obvious problem associated with the creation of a boney defect and

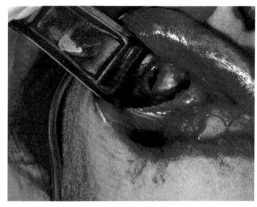

Fig. 12. Erosion of a cheek implant into the maxillary sinus is shown. Fortunately, this is a rare occurrence and most often a result of inadvertent entry during placement over a thin boney sinus wall.

potential damage to underlying structures like tooth roots, but it also leads to loss of chin projection.

It is commonly accepted that contemporary anatomic malar and chin implants cause some resorption, but the resorption is minimal and self-limiting. Boney erosion probably occurs less with anatomic extended implants because of greater distribution of the pressure forces over a broader anatomic area. Most studies report a 40%–60% incidence of some kind of erosion, but it is uncommon to have significant enough erosion to cause decreased chin projection.[30] Resorption appears to occur in the first 12 months after placement but can appear radiographically in as soon as 2 months.

In a retrospective study by Friedland and colleagues[31] of 85 silicone chin implants, the researchers found that up to 50% demonstrated some kind of absorbtion. They found that larger implants seemed to cause more absorption and felt that this was because of increases in local pressure due primarily to size and volume. In Hinderer's experience of placing over 1200 alloplastic facial implants, he recognized no major change in soft tissue contour due to underlying bone resorption. In the chin, he felt the results were due to avoiding placement over the thinner alveolar bone more superiorly.[32]

Significant bone resorption is rarely associated with malar implants. The rarity of resorption is thought to be due to the large surface contact relative to the size of the bone and the laxity of the soft tissue with minimal muscle pull against the bone. In Brennan's retrospective study of 10 patients followed up 2–4 years post placement of malar implants, he saw no radiographic evidence of maxillary bone resorption.[33]

Matrasso and colleagues theorize that particular patients are predisposed to exaggerated boney resorption under chin implants. This includes patients with labial incompetence who will overwork their mentalis. These patients typically have a long lower facial third with a class II dentoskeletal relation. Mentalis hyperactivity leads to pressure and migration of the implant superiorly onto the thinner bone of the alveolus, which predisposes to resorption. In their retrospective study of six patients undergoing orthognathic surgery who had previously had silastic implants placed and removed, 100% of the patients exhibited lip incompetence before surgery. Thus, the researchers contend that mentalis hyperactivity is a contraindication for genial implant placement. Additionally, implants are more likely to be placed higher on the chin in these patients for aesthetic purposes. This would also predispose them to resorption.

Under conditions of sever resorption, the implant must be removed. Removal of a chin implant can result in bizarre chin configurations with dimpling. Matrasso and colleagues advocate a horizontal genioplasty every time a chin implant is removed to diminish adverse sequela before soft tissue scarification and deformity.

Postoperative Asymmetry

Asymmetry is more likely to be noticed in malar implants because they are closer to the focal point of the face and obviously there is one placed bilaterally. Asymemetry is a major cause of patient dissatisfaction. Asymmetry has many causes, but it is usually caused by initial malposition or by creation of asymmetric bilaterally dissected spaces. It can also be the result of unrecognized preoperative skeletal or soft tissue deficiencies, which are present in up to 50% of the population preoperatively. It is important to point out preexisting asymmetry before treatment selection and treat these patients appropriately by using different size implants when necessary and different zonal placements.

Yarmechuck[34] reported on placement of 370 implants over the facial skeleton, with a 10 percent reoperation rate to improve symmetry and contour, primarily at the malar eminence. He attributed his success to subperiosteal placement and fixation with titanium screws as well as in place implant contouring.

Although major asymmetries require a second surgery, minor asymmetries have a natural tendency to adjust and correct themselves over a 6-month postoperative period as healing progresses and the tissue around the implant relaxes and softens.

Revision

Should a chin implant need to be removed, some surgeons feel that the remaining capsule will often provide adequate residual augmentation. As defined by Cohen and colleagues, removal of chin implants is not without morbidity. They evaluated ten patients who presented for treatment of chin deformities status post multiple attempts at augmentation and removal for migration or size discrepancies. They noted pogonial bunching and dimpling in repose or on animation in 90% of patients; asymmetric lower lip motion in 50%; and pain and tenderness on palpation in 20%. Their postulation was that de-gloving of the mentalis and the depressor labii inferioris displace the muscle origins. As the implant is placed and heals, the muscles redrape on the capsule. Thus, if the implant is removed, centripetal contraction occurs of the capsule with the muscle attachment thus causing the deformity. 40% patients sought surgical correction, which consisted of advancement genioplasty and resuspension of the mentalis. The researchers subsequent recommendations are that correcting residual skin dimpling is difficult and capsulectomy is a consideration, but prophylactic simultaneous genioplasty should be performed on all patients who require removal of their implants.[35]

As reported by Terino, revision operations carry a greater risk for nerve or muscle damage. This occurs as high as 30%–50% in his experience. This finding is understandable when one considers that removing a porous implant may involve a cuff of surrounding tissue and, for nonporous implants, this could involve dissection through or around an implant capsule to accommodate a larger implant. This procedure obviously increases risk for damage. To avoid nerve or muscle damage during implant removal, try to only dissect with in the capsule and directly on the surface of the implant.

SUMMARY

There are many factors that determine the success of the surgical attempt at alloplastic facial augmentation including patient's health status and recipient tissue bed, the biomaterials properties, and the expertise offered by the surgeon. To mount any response to the implanted material, the host must be healthy, well-nourished, and possessing a functional immune system. Thus, chronic disease, protein or calorie malnourishment, therapy with steroids or other cytotoxic drugs, or poor regional perfusion will lead to an increased risk for failure. Factors that minimize inflammation will maximize biocompatibility and minimize failure. The bioresponse will be minimized by an implant that is: nontoxic; nonantigenic; sufficient enough porosity size to allow immune cell entry and to allow native tissue in growth. The material should be nonparticulate, resistant to fragmentation, and able to be fixated. The surgeon should use sound clinical judgment, thorough preoperative facial analysis, adherence to fundamental surgical principles, meticulous implant handling, avoidance of a contaminated operative field, and perioperative use of antibiotics.[36] In addition, the surgeon should ensure that the biomaterial is appropriately matched to the tissue plane with in which it will be implanted. He or she should make proper assessment of tissue quality, with emphasis on vascularity, adequate soft tissue coverage, and adequate adaption and fixation of the implant. Only through these measures will complications be avoided.

REFERENCES

1. Sclafani AP, Romo T. Biology and chemistry of facial implants. Facial Plast Surg 2000;16(1):3–6.
2. Eppley B. Alloplastic implantation. Plast Reconstr Surg 1999;104(6):1761–85.
3. Scales J, Winter G. Clinical considerations in the choice of materials for orthopedic internal devices. J Biomed Mater Res 1975;9:167–76.
4. Morehead JM, Holt GR. Soft tissue response to synthetic biomaterials. Otolaryngol Clin North Am 1994; 27:195–201.
5. Wilkinson TS. Complications in aesthetic malar augmentation. Plast Reconstr Surg 1983;71(3):643–9.
6. Terino EO. Alloplastic contouring in the malar-midface-middle third facial aesthetic unit. In: Terino EO, Flowers RR, editors. The art of alloplastic facial contouring. St. Louis (MO): Mosby; 2000. p. 79–96.
7. Constanntinides MS, Galli SD, Miller PJ, et al. Malar submalar, and midfacial implants. Facial Plast Surg 2000;16(1):35–44.
8. Jabaley ME, Hoopes JE, Cochran TC. Transoral silastic augmentation of the malar region. Br J Plast Surg 1974;27:98–102.
9. Gross EJ, Hamilton MM, Ackermann K. Mersilene mesh chin augmentation. Arch Facial Plast Surg 1999;1:183–9.
10. Scaccia FJ, Allphin A, Stepnick DW. Complications of augmentation mentoplasty: a review of 11,095 cases. Int J Aesth Rest Surg 1983;1(1):3–8.
11. Roy D, Mangat DS. Facial implants. Dermatol Clin 2005;23(3):541–7.
12. Rubin JP, Yaremchuk MJ. Complications and toxicity of implantable biomaterials used in facial reconstructive and aesthetic surgery: a comprehensive review of the literature. Plast Reconstr Surg 1997; 100(5):1336–53.
13. Hasson O, Levi G, Conley R. Late infections associated with alloplastic facial implants. J Oral Maxillofac Surg 2007;65(2):321–3.
14. Yarmechuck MJ. Mandibular augmentation. Plast Reconstr Surg 2000;106(3):697–706.
15. Erlich MA, Parhiscar A. Nasal dorsal augmentation with silicone implants. Facial Plast Surg 2003; 19(4):325–30.
16. Jung DH, Kim BR, Choi JY, et al. Gross and pathologic analysis of long term silicone implants inserted into the human body for augmentation rhinoplasty: 221 revision cases. Plast Reconstr Surg 2007;120(7): 1997–2003.
17. Deva AK, Merton S, Chang L. Silicone in nasal augmentation rhinoplasty: a decade of clinical experience. Plast Reconstr Surg 1998;102(4):1230–7.
18. Metzinger SE, McCollough EG, Campbell JP, et al. Malar augmentation: a 5 year retrospective review of the silastic midface malar implant. Arch Otolaryngol Head Neck Surg 1999;125(9):980–7.
19. Terino EO. Chin and malar augmentation. In: Complications and problems in aesthetic plastic surgery. New York: NY; 1992. Ch 6.
20. Yarmechuck MJ. Infraorbital rim augmentation. Plast Reconstr Surg 2001;107(6):1585–92.
21. Sclafani AP, Thomas JR, Cox AJ, et al. Clinical and histologic response of subcutaneous expanded polytetraflouroethylene and porous high density polyethylene implants to acute and early infection. Arch Otolaryngol Head Neck Surg 1997;123: 328–36.
22. Zimmerli W, Waldvogel FA, Vaudaux P, et al. Pathogenesis of foreign body infection: description and characteristics of an animal model. J Infect Dis 1982;486(4):487–97.
23. Cohen SR, Kawamoto HK. Infection of proplast malar implants following dental injections. Plast Reconstr Surg 1992;89(6):1148–51.
24. Karras SC, Wolford LM. Augmentation genioplasty with hard tissue replacement implants. J Oral Maxillofac Surg 1998;56(5):549–52.
25. Louis PJ, Cuzalina LA. Alloplastic augmentation of the face. Atlas Oral Maxillofac Surg Clin North Am 2000; 8(2):127–91.
26. Constantino PD, Friedman CD, Lane A. Synthetic biomaterials in facial plastic and reconstructive surgery. Facial Plast Surg 1993;9(1):1–15.
27. Frodel JL, Lee S. The use of high density polyethylene implants in facial deformities. Arch Otolaryngol Head Neck Surg 2007;124(11):1219–23.
28. Whitaker LA. Aesthetic augmentation of the malar midface structures. Plast Reconstr Surg 1987; 80(2):337–46.
29. Robinson M. Bone resorption under plastic chin implants. Arch Otolaryngol 1972;95(1):30–3.

30. Matarasso A, Elias AC, Elias R. Labial incompetence: a marker for progressive bone resorption in silastic chin augmentation. Plast Reconstr Surg 1996;98(6):1007–14.

31. Friedland JA, Coccaro PJ, Converse JM. Retospective cephalometric analysis of mandibular bone absorption under silicone rubber chin implants. Plast Reconstr Surg 1976;57(20):144–51.

32. Hinderer UT. Nasal base maxillary and infraorbital implants-alloplastic. Clin Plast Surg 1991;18(1):87–101.

33. Brennan HG. Augmentation malarplasty. Arch Otolaryngol 1982;108(7):441–4.

34. Yaremchuck MJ. Facial skeletal reconstruction using porous polyethylene implants. Plast Reconstr Surg 2003;111(6):1818–27.

35. Cohen SR, Mardach OL, Kawawmoto HK. Chin disfigurement following removal of alloplastic chin implants. Plast Reconstr Surg 1991;88(1):62–7.

36. Zim S. Skeletal volume enhancement: implants and osteotomies. Curr Opin Otolaryngol Head Neck Surg 2004;12(4):349–56.

Otoplasty Complications

Todd G. Owsley, DDS, MD*, Teresa G. Biggerstaff, DDS, MD

KEYWORDS

- Otoplasty • Complications • Diagnosis
- Prevention • Treatment

Otoplasty, the correction of protruding ears, is a commonly performed cosmetic surgical procedure. It is a procedure that can produce significant patient and surgeon satisfaction. Affecting 5% of the population, prominent or protruding ears are a common congenital anomaly. Correcting this problem at an early age can prevent ridicule from peers and enhance self-esteem. Although most cosmetic surgical procedures are performed on adults, otoplasty is most commonly performed on children.

Although they are few and rare, otoplasty has associated risks and complications. Most of these complications can be minimized by appropriate patient selection, careful preoperative analysis and planning, meticulous surgical technique, and compliant postoperative care. The surgeon must be familiar with the possible complications to avoid or prevent them. The astute surgeon must also be able to recognize and confidently treat adverse outcomes as they occur to minimize long-term sequelae.

SURGICAL TECHNIQUES

More than 170 surgical techniques are described in the literature to correct protruding ears. This article addresses the more commonly performed techniques and the associated related complications. The two deformities that most commonly occur in patients with protruding ears can occur either individually or in combination. The first is a poorly developed antihelical fold (**Fig. 1**). Without an antihelical fold, the ear lacks definition between the conchal bowl and the scapha. This results in excessive lateral projection of the upper portion of the helix. In a normal ear the concha-scapha angle approximates 90 degrees (**Fig. 2**). If the

antihelical fold is absent or weak it may measure up to 150 degrees. The second abnormality involves the formation of excessive conchal cartilage, particularly in the posterior conchal wall (**Fig. 3**). Conchal bowl hypertrophy causes excessive protrusion of the auricle away from the scalp in the middle and lower portions of the ear. The ideal ear demonstrates an auriculocephalic (AC) angle of 30 degrees (see **Fig. 2**). With conchal hypertrophy this angle may approach 45 degrees. Other deformities include a protruding earlobe, helical rim deformities, and anteromedially displaced insertion of the postauricular muscle.[1] It is important to recognize the cause of the protruding ear in order to select the appropriate surgical technique or techniques for correction.

Many techniques address conchal bowl hypertrophy. These techniques can be classified as cartilage-cutting or cartilage-sparing techniques. The most commonly used cartilage-cutting technique that addresses conchal hypertrophy is the Davis technique. The Davis technique involves excising the hypertrophic portion of the posterior conchal wall through a postauricular incision (**Fig. 4**). This allows a passive correction, bringing the ear to a more normal position in relation to the scalp.[1] The most common cartilage-sparing technique is the Furnas technique, which involves placing conchomastoid sutures through a postauricular incision.[2]

Techniques that address the lack of an antihelical fold are classified as "suture-only" or scoring techniques. Mustarde described recreating the antihelical fold by placing conchoscaphal horizontal mattress sutures (**Fig. 5**). The Stenstrom technique involves scoring the anterior surface of the scapha and relying on cartilage bending away from the weakened cartilage as it heals to recreate

Carolina Surgical Arts, 2516 Oakcrest Avenue, Suite B, Greensboro, NC 27408, USA
* Corresponding author.
E-mail address: tgowsley@csagso.com (T.G. Owsley).

Oral Maxillofacial Surg Clin N Am 21 (2009) 105–118
doi:10.1016/j.coms.2008.10.011
1042-3699/08/$ – see front matter © 2009 Elsevier Inc. All rights reserved.

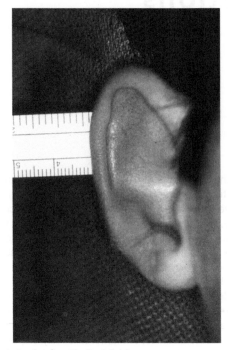

Fig. 2. An axial section at the level of the helical crus demonstrates the ideal auriculocephalic angle (AC) of 30 degrees. (*Modified from* Tanzer RC. Congenital deformities. In: Converse J, editor. Reconstructive plastic surgery. 2nd edition. Philadelphia: WB Saunders; 1977. p. 1710; with permission.)

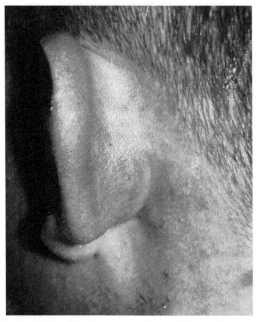

Fig. 1. Lack of antihelical fold.

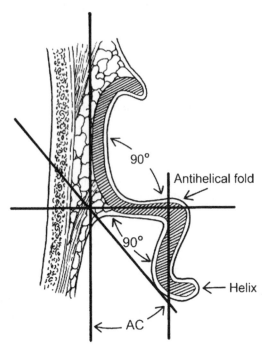

Fig. 3. Conchal bowl hypertrophy.

the antihelical fold. These techniques are often used in combination with a conchal setback procedure.

POSTOPERATIVE HEMORRHAGE AND HEMATOMA

The blood supply to the external ear is extensive. The arterial blood supply to the ear is derived from the superficial temporal artery and the posterior auricular artery, both branches of the external carotid artery. The superficial temporal artery emerges 1 cm anterior to the ear and deep to the anterior auricular muscle. It divides into superior, medial, and inferior branches that supply the anterior and anterolateral surface of the auricle. The posterior auricular artery travels parallel to the postauricular crease and crosses deep to the great auricular nerve and the posterior auricular muscle. Knowledge of this anatomy is important to avoid damage to these arteries during surgery.[1]

Because of this extensive blood supply with numerous perforating vessels through the cartilage, the ear is able to tolerate multiple surgical approaches simultaneously. The abundant blood supply can also contribute, however, to postoperative bleeding and hematoma.

During otoplastic surgery, overzealous use of epinephrine can cause bleeding because of a rebound effect from the vasoconstrictor.[3–5] To

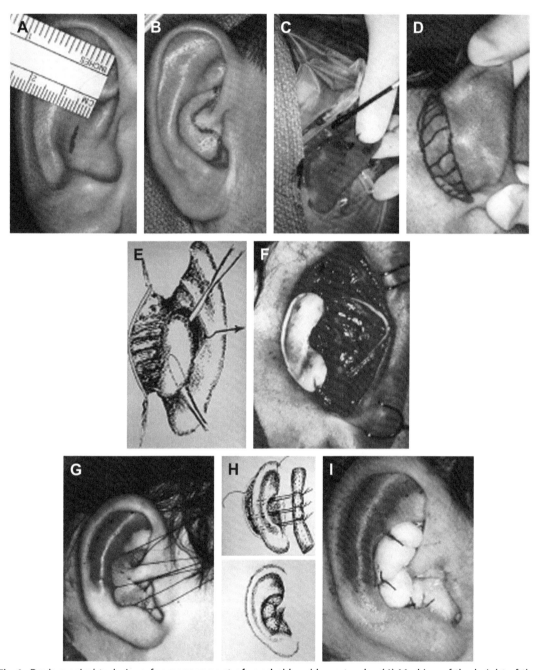

Fig. 4. Davis surgical technique for management of conchal bowl hypertrophy. (*A*) Marking of the height of the posterior conchal wall that will remain. (*B*) Marking the conchal bowl to be excised. (*C*) Transferring the marking to the underlying cartilage with methylene blue. (*D*) Initial amount of skin to be removed in an elliptic fashion. (*E, F*) Postauricular view of excised cartilage. (*G–I*) Through-and-through fixation sutures anchored to postauricular muscle and mastoid fascia used to secure cotton bolster. (*E, H From* Davis JE. Prominent ears. Clin Plast Surg 1978;5:475; *A–D, F, G, I From* Owsley TG. Otoplastic surgery for the protruding ear. In: Fonseca RJ, editor. Oral and maxillofacial surgery. Philadelphia: WB Saunders; 2000. p. 415; with permission.)

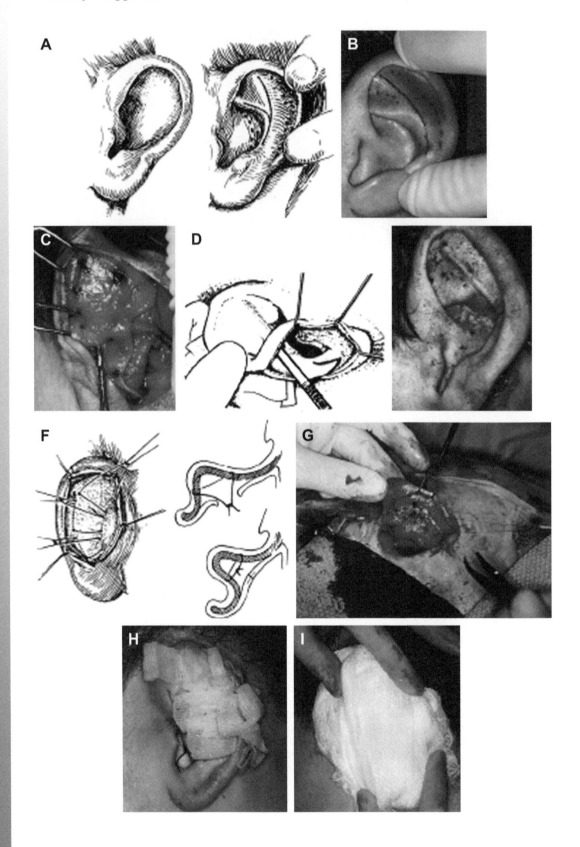

prevent this, local anesthetic with 1:100,000 epinephrine should be used judiciously.[5] Meticulous dissection during the operation can result in a nearly bloodless field, whereas dissection in inappropriate planes can cause bleeding and hematoma formation. Electrocautery also should be used during surgery to achieve hemostasis. Calder and Naasan[6] reported a 2% incidence of postoperative bleeding or hematoma. Most of these cases can be attributed to inadequate hemostasis during surgery.[6–8] Goode and coworkers[9] reported a 3.5% incidence of hematoma, two cases of which were caused by postoperative trauma. Weerda and Siegert[10] recommend use of a drain for 24 hours postoperatively to help prevent this complication.

Hematoma can also result from an occult coagulopathy. As with any surgery, a complete and detailed preoperative medical history should be obtained.

The cardinal signs of postoperative hematoma are excessive pain, a tense bluish swelling more commonly in the postauricular area, and a blood-soaked dressing within the initial 24 hours (**Fig. 6**). Otoplasty patients should be examined within 24 hours following surgery to recognize signs of bleeding and hematoma formation.

Once a hematoma has been diagnosed, it should be treated promptly with removal of the clot, simple drainage, antibiotics, and a compression dressing (**Fig. 7**). If there is evidence of ongoing bleeding, exploration of the surgical site with meticulous hemostasis is necessary. If a hematoma is not recognized or if treatment is delayed, it can lead to necrosis of the skin (**Fig. 8**) or cartilage, infection, and formation of cauliflower ear deformity.

In surgery, simple steps can be followed to prevent these complications:

1. Obtain a detailed medical history and physical exam before surgery
2. Judicious use of local anesthetic with epinephrine
3. Meticulous dissection
4. Diligent hemostasis with electrocautery intraoperatively
5. Closure of the incisions only after a dry field is obtained
6. Precise placement of a compression dressing
7. Close follow-up postoperatively
8. Instructions to avoid trauma to the ear in the postoperative period

INFECTION

Infection following otoplasty is rare with a reported incidence of 2.4% to 5.2%.[6,9] If an infection occurs, it can lead to perichondritis with loss of cartilage and a devastating residual deformity of the ear. The most common organisms responsible for postoperative infections of the ear include *Staphylococcus*, *Streptococcus*, and more rarely *Pseudomonas aeruginosa* and *Escherichia coli*.[9,11] Most infections occur greater than 5 days postoperatively.[9]

Signs of postoperative infection include wound erythema, discharge, prolonged edema, and pain. When infection is suspected, a wound culture and sensitivity should be obtained and the patient should be treated with the appropriate antibiotics.[10,12] If purulence is recognized, the operative site is drained, irrigated, and any suture material is removed. Necrotic skin or cartilage should be debrided (**Fig. 9**).

Appropriate preoperative skin preparation of the patient, strict sterile technique, perioperative antibiotics, and local wound care are paramount in avoiding infections. A single dose of an intravenous broad-spectrum antibiotic, such as cefazolin, should be given before the incision. The sterile preparation of the operative site should include the hair around the ear, the external ear, and the external auditory meatus. The external auditory meatus should be protected during the procedure with an ointment-moistened cotton ball. The closed incision should be coated with a triple antibiotic ointment. Postoperative antibiotics that cover *Pseudomonas*, such as ciprofloxacin, should be considered.

Patient selection can affect the rate of postoperative infection after otoplasty. Patients with postauricular eczema are more prone to infection after otoplasty because of the increased

Fig. 5. Mustarde surgical technique for creating antihelical fold. (*A, B*) Creating and marking the desired antihelical fold by folding back the helix with digital pressure. Lines, parallel to the crest of the fold, are marked and transferred to the underlying cartilage and used to guide suture placement. (*C–E*) Dissection of the scaphoid fossa beneath the anterior skin for weakening and creation of the desired antihelical fold. (*F, G*) Placement of horizontal mattress sutures to create a new antihelical fold. (*H, I*) Placement of petrolatum gauze and fluffs as an important pressure dressing. (*A, F From* La Trenta GS. Otoplasty. In: Rees TD, La Trenta GS, editors. Aesthetic plastic surgery. 2nd edition. Philadelphia: WB Saunders; 1995; *D Modified from* Stenstrom SJ, Heftner JL. The Stenstrom otoplasty. Clin Plast Surg 1978;5:467; *B, C, E, G, H, I From* Owsley TG. Otoplastic surgery for the protruding ear. In: Fonseca RJ, editor. Oral and maxillofacial surgery. Philadelphia: WB Saunders; 2000. p. 417; with permission.)

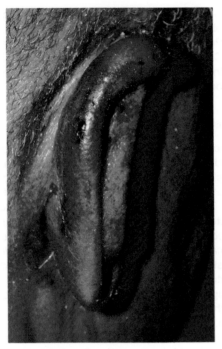

Fig. 6. Postauricular hematoma after using Mustarde sutures for creation of antihelical fold.

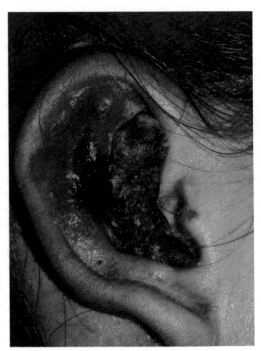

Fig. 8. Anterior skin necrosis secondary to anterior hematoma. (*Courtesy of* Joseph Niamtu, DMD, Richmond, VA.)

colonization of *Staphylococcus aureus* in eczematous skin.[11] Otoplasty should be delayed until eczema around the ears resolves. Surgery should also be delayed in any patients with otitis externa.[9]

KELOID AND HYPERTROPHIC SCARRING

Adverse scarring is rare following otoplasty. When it does occur, it can be a difficult problem to manage. Excessive proliferation of normal healing tissue results in both hypertrophic scars and keloids. Hypertrophic scars and keloids are included in the spectrum of fibroproliferative disorders. These scars result from the loss of control mechanisms that regulate the balance between tissue repair and tissue regeneration. The postauricular incision is especially susceptible to adverse scarring because of the sparse population of sebaceous glands.

Hypertrophic scarring refers to excessive scarring that occurs within the confines of the original incision or scar line. These scars are typically raised, erythematous, and fibrotic. They usually occur within the first few months of the initial surgery and remain stable or regress over time. Hypertrophic scarring may be related to excessive postauricular skin excision necessitating wound closure under tension. This can be avoided by planning a conservative elliptic excision of skin or delaying the skin excision until the completion of

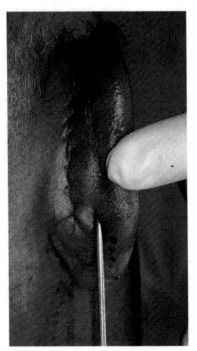

Fig. 7. Drain placement after evacuation of hematoma.

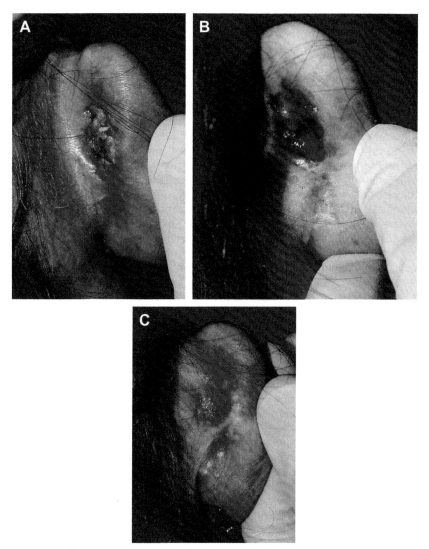

Fig. 9. (*A*) Postauricular infection with extrusion of suture material. (*B*) Suture removed and area debrided. (*C*) Postauricular infection site healed. (*Courtesy of* Joseph Niamtu, DMD, Richmond, VA.)

the procedure. To avoid overexcision of skin, the postauricular skin can be left without an elliptic excision. This can leave some skin redundancy, but the pleating flattens and resolves over time.

Keloid scarring refers to excessive scarring that extends beyond the original incision or scar line. Keloids occasionally cause pain, itching, and paresthesia. Darker pigmented patients are at a greater risk for keloids, especially if they have a personal or family history of keloids. If a patient reports a personal history of keloid scarring it is especially important to close the incision passively. It may be prudent to inject the incision line with a steroid as it heals. Steroid injections act by decreasing collagen synthesis, decreasing mucinous ground substance, and inhibiting collagenase inhibitors that prevent the breakdown of collagen

(which decreases dermal thickening). Injection of the steroid should be into the papillary dermis. Typically, triamcinolone is used and is available in 10 mg/mL or 40 mg/mL. Injections should be performed every 4 to 6 weeks for a total of 6 months to prevent keloid formation.

If treating an existing keloid, the size of the keloid determines the amount of steroid to be injected. This author uses approximately 0.2 mL of 40 mg/mL triamcinolone per centimeter of keloid. These injections are repeated every 3 to 6 weeks until the scar has flattened sufficiently. If the steroid injections prove to be insufficient treatment, the keloid can be excised. After excision steroid injections should commence and continue at 4- to 6-week intervals for 6 months to prevent recurrence. Drawbacks to intralesional injection of steroids include possible depigmentation, hyper-pigmentation, or tissue atrophy. In children, intra-lesional steroid injections are not well-tolerated secondary to pain. Golladay[13] advocates a single intraoperative injection of betamethasone acetate at the time of keloid excision and reports only one recurrence in 28 cases.

Other methods of treating keloids include radia-tion treatment following excision, pressure dress-ings, silicone dressings, and cryosurgery. A typical radiation regimen starts the day of surgery and involves 300 Gy every other day for 4 days or 500 Gy every day for 3 days. Radiation when com-bined with excision of keloids has shown a preven-tion of recurrence in 80% to 94% of cases. Shielding of the adjacent areas is prudent to pre-vent other associated complications with irradia-tion. Children should not be irradiated unless it is the only viable option. Specialized pressure dress-ings that provide compression of the scar have been shown to be effective in the treatment of ke-loids. The postauricular area is an awkward and difficult place to treat with a compression dress-ing. The mechanism of action of pressure dress-ings is unknown. One theory is that by occluding small blood vessels there is a reduction in tissue metabolism, fibroblast proliferation, and collagen synthesis. Cryosurgery is the use of liquid nitrogen to "freeze" the lesion. Regimens include one to three freeze cycles lasting from 10 to 30 seconds, repeated every 20 to 30 days. Cryotherapy when used in combination with intralesional steroids has a reported success rate of 84% (significant flattening and no recurrence). One of the main ad-vantages of using cryotherapy is that it causes little to no pain during treatment;[14] the downside is that results can be unpredictable.

TELEPHONE EAR AND REVERSE TELEPHONE EAR

Residual deformity of the ear following otoplasty is one of the more common complications. Tele-phone ear occurs when there is overcorrection of the middle one third of the conchal bowl (**Fig. 10**). The middle portion of the conchal bowl lies closer to the scalp if overcorrected. This gives the appearance of protruding superior and inferior poles. Telephone ear deformity can also result from undercorrection of the superior and inferior poles. Reverse telephone ear occurs when there is overcorrection of the superior and inferior poles of the ear, or undercorrection of the middle third. These complications are easily avoided by careful preoperative planning and proper intraoperative technique.

Crucial preoperative measurements include the distance that the helix is from the scalp at the superior pole, at the inferior pole, and at the widest portion of the helix over the mastoid. In an ideal ear the superior aspect of the helix should be 10 mm from the scalp. The widest portion of the helix should be 18 to 20 mm from the scalp over the mastoid.[10] These ideal numbers should assist the surgeon during the operation and intraoperative measurements should be taken to ensure the best result. If the patient requires both recreation of the antihelical fold and conchal setback, the conchal setback should be performed first. An-other aspect of an esthetic ear to consider when performing otoplasty is that when viewing the ear from the frontal view the helical rim should be vis-ible just lateral to the prominence of the antihelix. Positioning the patient during surgery to be able to evaluate the ear from the frontal view is crucial in obtaining a good result and is helpful in achiev-ing symmetry with the opposite ear.

SUTURE COMPLICATIONS

Commonly used techniques for correcting a prom-inent ear include the Mustarde technique for recre-ating an antihelical fold and the Furnas technique for decreasing prominence of the conchal bowl. Both of these techniques use permanent sutures to maintain the new position of the ear. Several complications can arise because of these suturing techniques or the type of suture used. These

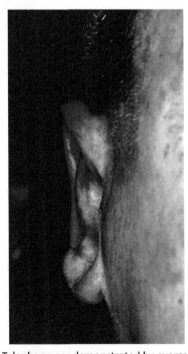

Fig. 10. Telephone ear demonstrated by overcorrection of middle third of ear.

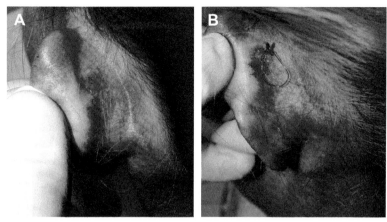

Fig. 11. (*A*) Extrusion of permanent monofilament suture material with no surrounding infection. (*B*) Removal of suture. (*Courtesy of* Joseph Niamtu, DMD, Richmond, VA.)

complications include surface irregularities, erosion of the sutures through the skin, contour irregularities of the ear, narrowing of the external auditory meatus, bowstringing, and granuloma formation (**Figs. 11** and **12**).

Monofilament nonabsorbable sutures, such as nylon or polypropylene, can erode through the thin postauricular skin causing suture fistulae or granuloma formation. Polyfilament nonabsorbable sutures, such as silk or polyester, may cause less erosion through the skin, but tend to have a higher infection risk.[4]

Bowstringing, or visible bridging of sutures beneath the thin postauricular skin, can be caused by any type of permanent suture. It occurs because of placing sutures under tension across a gap spanning an area with little to no subcutaneous tissue. In most cases, bowstringing is tolerated by the patient and requires no treatment. When sutures erode or cause granulomas, however, they

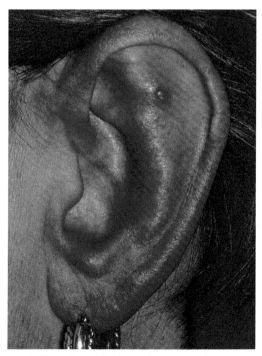

Fig. 12. Extrusion of Mustarde suture (permanent monofilament) through anterior skin.

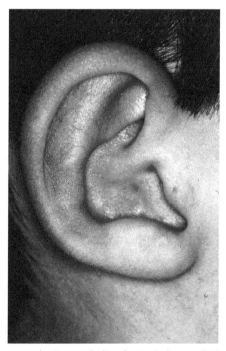

Fig. 13. Esthetic antihelix formed by well-placed Mustarde sutures.

need to be removed. Sutures can safely be removed after 6 months without fear of relapse.

The author prefers using 4–0 mersilene suture for the Mustarde technique. The postauricular skin incision is closed with 4–0 plain gut suture. Plain gut suture is less likely to incite a local inflammatory response or granuloma formation, as can be seen with subcuticular polyglactin or polyglycolic acid suture.

ANTIHELICAL DEFORMITIES

Anterior scoring and rasping techniques may be necessary when utilizing the Mustarde technique, especially in patients with thick and noncompliant cartilage. This roughening of the antihelix may result in visible irregularities along the scapha and along the prominence of the antihelix. The Stenstrom technique requires extensive anterior dissection. The extensive undermining leaves this area prone to hematoma and necrosis of the skin. The cartilage incisions in this technique may also leave anterior irregularities visible through the thin anterior skin.

When placing Mustarde sutures it is important to remember that an esthetic antihelix has a gentle curve (**Fig. 13**). To ensure accurate creation of an esthetic curved antihelix, the desired location of the fold should be marked on the anterior surface of the ear. Marks are then placed parallel to the planned crest of the fold at least 7 mm apart to avoid creating too narrow of a fold. The lateral marks are then transferred to the underlying cartilage with a hypodermic needle dipped in methylene blue.[1] Sutures should be placed perpendicularly across the antihelical fold, so that on tightening, a well-round antihelix is created. The sutures should be placed in a radial fashion rather than in a straight line to create the natural appearing antihelical fold.

Conchal Bowl Deformities

Excising a portion of the conchal bowl, if not done meticulously, can cause deformities that are visible through the anterior skin. This "injury" to the conchal cartilage may result in abnormal cartilage growth (**Fig. 14**). Rough cartilage edges at the periphery of the excision may show through the thin anterior skin (**Fig. 15**). Hyperpigmentation of the anterior skin can result from placement of the conchal bowl dressing (**Fig. 16**). If dissection planes are not carefully maintained, the anterior skin may be perforated during conchal bowl excision (**Fig. 17**).

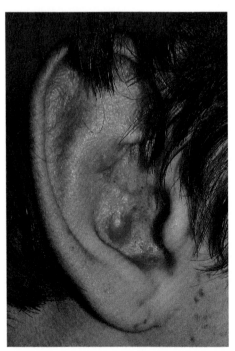

Fig. 14. Abnormal cartilage growth after conchal bowl excision.

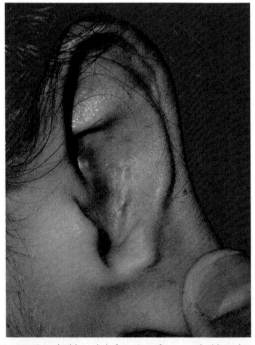

Fig. 15. Conchal bowl deformity after conchal bowl excision; rough edge is visible through anterior skin. (*Courtesy of* Joseph Niamtu, DMD, Richmond, VA.)

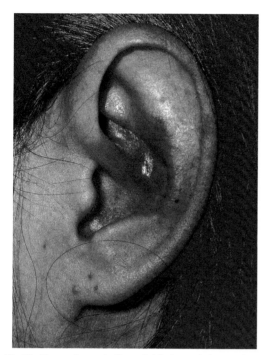

Fig. 16. Hyperpigmentation of skin in an Asian patient.

Earlobe Deformities

A protruding earlobe often accompanies a protruding ear. A common mistake when correcting protruding ears is to disregard the earlobes. The surgeon can obtain disappointing results if close attention is not paid to the position of the earlobes during otoplastic surgery. Typically, patients with protruding ears have a cauda helicis (helical tail),

which protrudes laterally. Some surgeons try to compensate for this by simply excising postauricular skin and obliterating the postauricular sulcus. This may provide temporary improvement, but over time the correction is lost. Instead, in these patients, the helical tail should be addressed directly. Through the postauricular incision the helical tail can be identified. A cauda-conchal mattress suture is then placed to draw in the lobe the desired amount.[12,15]

Skin excision may be necessary to correct any residual deformity at this point. This is done by extending the postauricular incision in a fishtail fashion and excising the redundant skin (**Figs. 18 and 19**).

NARROWING OF THE EXTERNAL AUDITORY MEATUS

Conchal setback without cartilage excision is prone to causing narrowing of the external auditory meatus and occasionally can cause complete occlusion. This complication is more common in adult ears, which tend to have thicker, less flexible cartilage. With the Furnas technique of conchal setback an excellent cosmetic result can be obtained. In tacking the conchal cartilage to the mastoid periosteum, however, the natural spring of the cartilage places the anterior lip of the conchal bowl into the external auditory meatus (**Fig. 20**).[16,17] Furnas attributes this problem to poor placement of the conchal-mastoid sutures. If using this technique the ear should be repositioned posteriorly and medially to prevent narrowing of the ear canal.[12] Another solution to this potential problem

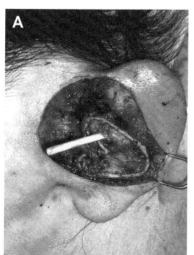
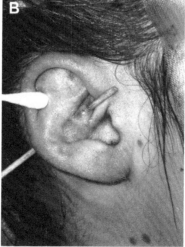

Fig. 17. Perforation of anterior skin during conchal bowl excision. (*Courtesy of* Joseph Niamtu, DMD, Richmond, VA.)

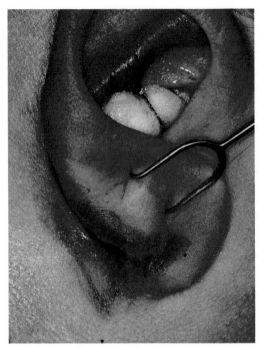

Fig. 18. Fishtail excision for correction of prominent earlobe. Posterior aspect of excision is planned by outlining anterior aspect of excision with a surgical marker, then transferring this marking to skin posterior to earlobe.

is to excise a small ellipse of meatal cartilage through the postauricular incision.[16]

RELAPSE

Relapse of an ear deformity is a disappointing complication that may not become evident until months after surgery. Relapse can occur because of a variety of reasons. Using resorbable suture material for key portions of the procedure, such as Mustarde sutures, may show temporary correction, but over time weakens and resorbs and results in relapse (**Figs. 21–23**). Permanent suture materials may loosen or "slip" over time. They may also erode through the cartilage. Cartilage-scoring techniques can be unpredictable, especially in ears with thick and noncompliant cartilage.

If using the Furnas technique for conchal setback the surgeon must be certain to anchor the sutures firmly in both the conchal cartilage and the mastoid periosteum to prevent loss of correction. Some surgeons advocate slight overcorrection at the time of surgery to allow for rebound of the cartilage.

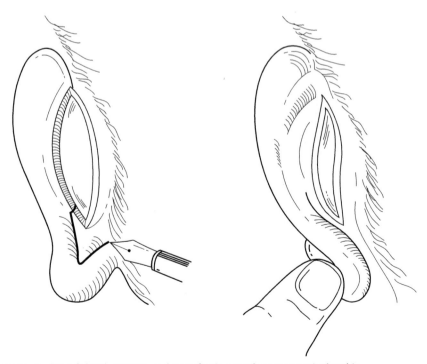

Fig. 19. Schematic marking fishtail excision and transferring mark to postauricular skin.

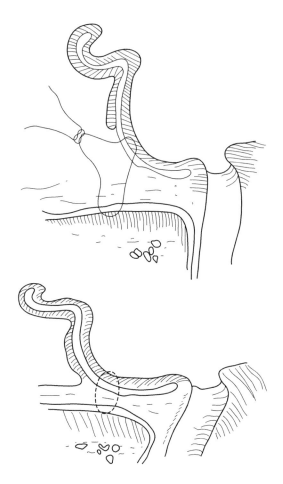

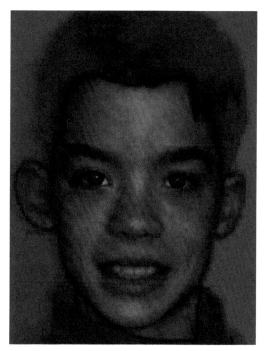

Fig. 21. Preoperative photo demonstrating prominent right ear caused by lack of antihelical fold and conchal bowl hypertrophy.

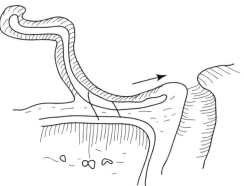

Fig. 20. Narrowing of the external auditory meatus because of rotation of the anterior lip of conchal bowl when using Furnas technique.

SUMMARY

Fortunately, otoplastic surgery carries few complications. As with all cosmetic surgical procedures, proper patient selection is imperative. Accurate preoperative assessment and the appropriate choice of a surgical correction can minimize unfavorable results. It is important to have a working

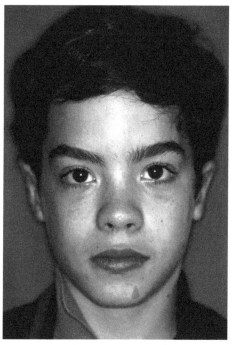

Fig. 22. Four months postoperative after right ear correction using Davis technique and Mustarde technique. Good correction still evident.

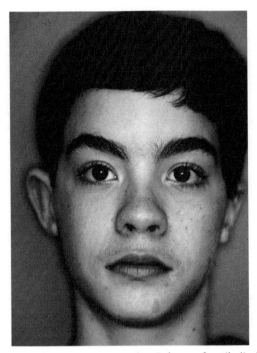

Fig. 23. One year postoperative. Relapse of antihelical correction (Mustarde sutures) caused by use of resorbable suture material.

knowledge of the potential complications of otoplasty and their prevention and treatment.

REFERENCES

1. Owsley TG. Otoplastic surgery for the protruding ear. Atlas Oral Maxillofac Surg Clin North Am 2004; 12(1):131–9.
2. Furnas DW. Otoplasty for prominent ears. Clin Plast Surg 2002;29(1):273–88.
3. Goodwin MR. Pitfalls in otoplasty. Eye Ear Nose Throat Mon 1970;49(1):4–6.
4. Furnas DW. Complications of surgery of the external ear. Clin Plast Surg 1990;17(2):305–18.
5. Steal S, Klebuc M, Spira M. Otoplasty. In: Goldwyn RM, Cohen MN, editors. The unfavorable result in plastic surgery: avoidance and treatment. 3rd edition. Philadelphia: Lippincott Williams and Wilkins; 2001. p. 437–50.
6. Calder JC, Naasan A. Morbidity of otoplasty: a review of 562 consecutive cases. Br J Plast Surg 1994;47(3):170–4.
7. Burres S. The anterior-posterior otoplasty. Arch Otolaryngol Head Neck Surg 1998;124(2):181–5.
8. Richards SD, Jebreel A, Capper R. Otoplasty: a review of the surgical techniques. Clin Otolaryngol 2005;30(1):2–8.
9. Goode RL, Profitt SD, Rafaty FM. Complications of otoplasty. Arch Otolaryngol 1970;91(4):352–5.
10. Weerda H, Siegert R. Complications in otoplastic surgery and their treatment. Facial Plast Surg 1994;10(3):287–97.
11. Beckett KS, Gault DT. Operating in an eczematous surgical field: don't be rash, delay surgery to avoid infective complications. J Plast Reconstr Aesthet Surg 2006;59(12):1446–9.
12. Adamson PA. Complications of otoplasty. Ear Nose Throat J 1985;64(12):568–74.
13. Golladay ES. Treatment of keloids by single intraoperative perilesional injection of repository steroid. South Med J 1988;81(6):736–8.
14. Muti E, Ponzio E. Cryotherapy in the treatment of keloids. Ann Plast Surg 1983;11(3):227–32.
15. Goulian D, Conway H. Prevention of persistent deformity of the tragus and lobule by modification of the Luckett technique of otoplasty. Plast Reconstr Surg Transplant Bull 1960;26(1):399–404.
16. Small A. Prevention of meatal stenosis in conchal setback otoplasty. Laryngoscope 1975;85(10):1782–5.
17. Adamson PA, Litner JA. Otoplasty technique. Facial Plast Surg Clin North Am 2006;14(2):79–87.

Complications in Hair Restoration Surgery

David Perez-Meza, MD[a],*, Robert Niedbalski, DO[b]

KEYWORDS

- Hair transplant surgery • Complications
- Donor area • Recipient area
- Follicular unit transplantation • Scalp surgery
- Hair restoration surgery

Hair loss affects more than 1.2 billion people around the world. Widely acknowledged as the only permanent solution for male and female pattern of hair loss, hair transplant surgery (HTS) has seen a surge in popularity the last 12 to 15 years.[1–4] A 2005 International Society of Hair Restoration Surgery survey reported more than 165,000 HTS cases were performed in the United States and around the world.[5] The American Society of Plastic Surgery also reported 39,000 HTS surgery cases performed by their constituency during the same period of time. The combined procedure count of about 200,000 is a sharp increase when compared with previous years and is likely to continue trending upward as public awareness and acceptance increases for surgical hair restoration. As the number of surgeries continues to rise, so too will the total number of complications that occur in the course of these operations and beyond, presenting major challenges to novice and seasoned HTS surgeons alike (**Fig. 1**).

DEFINITION

A complication is an adverse event that is not considered to be a common or usual occurrence, and which requires a change in methodology. The surgeon and staff should be familiar with any aspect related to the surgery, including a possible complication.

Dealing with a complication is like having a snake's nest on top of one's head (**Fig. 2**). They are difficult to handle and require a great deal of expertise and patience to manage them in the best way possible. Every patient is unique

and medicine and surgery are not exact sciences, so a successful outcome requires two critical steps: planning and execution. Most surgeons agree that "complications" is not a preferred topic of conversation to have with patients or staff.[6] As such, the surgeon, the staff, and the patient should be familiar with the type of problems that might present themselves when HTS is undertaken. Taking the time to educate patients and staff about HTS complications is an essential part of the planning phase. The hair transplant surgeon is dependent not only on his or her skill, experience, and knowledge, and the relationship with the patient, but also on some variables that are out of one's control. Complications can occur despite the best trained and qualified surgeon or staff, without any negligence whatsoever on the part of the surgeon, staff, or patient. Sometimes the HTS outcome is excellent and natural but the patient is still unhappy or unsatisfied. The key to understanding this contradiction is in seeing the results through the patient's eyes. HTS is an elective procedure and has limitations that should be discussed in detail one or more times with the patient before proceeding. Taking the time properly to educate patients can bridge the gap between the surgeon's expectations and the patient's expectations. Surgeons also need to learn to say "no" to patients on occasion. If there is a difficult patient with too many red flags (cons), sometimes the best result is obtained when surgery is not performed at all.

The reality is that any surgeon who performs HTS may have a complication and he or she

[a] Private Practice (Plastic and Hair Transplant Surgery Center), Mexico City, Mexico
[b] Medical Hair Restoration, Bellevue, WA, USA
* Corresponding author. 602 Nicoma Trail, Maitland, FL 32751.
E-mail address: drdavid@perez-meza.com (D. Perez-Meza).

Oral Maxillofacial Surg Clin N Am 21 (2009) 119–148
doi:10.1016/j.coms.2008.10.010
1042-3699/08/$ – see front matter © 2009 Elsevier Inc. All rights reserved.

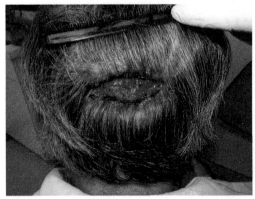

Fig. 1. Wound dehiscence of the donor area. Patient came for second opinion after 12 days postoperative (PO).

should aspire to prevent and resolve the complications. When a complication arises the surgeon should avoid some common mistakes. (1) Do not minimize the complication or worse yet, deny it even exists. Acknowledging the problem is the first step to resolving. (2) Do not antagonize an angry patient by arguing with them. Listen to their concerns and remain calm and supportive. (3) Do not be inaccessible to the patient. Be available for follow-up visits, telephone calls, emails, and so forth. Many times the complication can be resolve in a satisfactory way but the patient must receive and "feel" the physician's support to avoid ongoing problems.

This article provides an overview of the complications most likely to occur with modern hair restoration surgery (HRS) patients including hair transplant patients and scalp surgery, and more importantly provides recommendations on how to treat and prevent them in the first place. Corrections of HRS complications use different surgical techniques including single follicular or

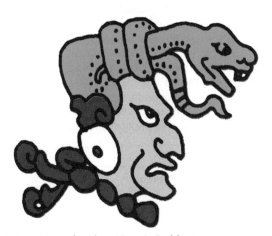

Fig. 2. Maya drawing, Moon's Goddess.

multifollicular unit, excision, forehead lift, tissue expanders, tissue extenders, and skin flaps. Hair restoration techniques used to correct or update old technology (hair plugs) is not within the scope of this article but is described elsewhere.[7–9]

INCIDENCE AND CLASSIFICATION

The incidence of complications in HRS is anecdotally much less than those encountered in other types of cosmetic procedures, but unfortunately no data are available to corroborate this information. In this article complications are divided into three categories corresponding to a familiar time: (1) preoperative, (2) intraoperative, and (3) postoperative.[10]

Preoperative

In the preoperative period, there are many factors that influence the outcome of the surgery. There can be preoperative complications even before performing a surgery. If those factors are not evaluated adequately and the surgery is performed, the stage is set for complications to occur.

Patient selection criteria

A thorough consultation is essential in HTS. All aspects of the patient's hair loss and possible treatment options[11–14] should be discussed, including both medical and surgical options. During this process, special attention should be given to understanding the patient's expectations. Specifically, these expectations usually refer to the procedure itself (step-by-step description of the patient's day in the operating room) and the end result (what they will see in the mirror 1 year postoperative). It is often during these discussions that red flags emerge as to any disparity between the patient's expectations and what can be accomplished within the patient's (financial and donor) budget. Patients often want to restore their hair as it was before the hair loss started, without side effects or complications. In the perfect world this is what the surgeon also wants, but often the reality is somewhat different.

It must be kept in mind that hair loss is devastating for men, but generally causes more impact and psychologic problems in women. The patient also thinks that after HTS the changes will lead to a better quality of life or lifestyle. This underscores the importance of the initial consultation as an integral part of the HRS process. Patient selection is a priority and just as important to the end result as selecting the right surgical technique.[15]

The surgeon must be honest with the patient during the consultation. They should know about the common complications that may occur and what steps will be taken if they do occur. The patient who undergoes HRS with such knowledge almost expects something to happen and is grateful if it does not occur. If the patient is not prepared for complications, however, they expect a surgery and postoperative course without any bumps in the road. Then, when problems do occur, the patient interprets the occurrence as lack of care on the part of the surgeon. If a patient has a complication from another surgeon, the situation should be dealt with as professionally as possible.

Use the consultation interview to look for personality disorders, such as body dysmorphic disorder, and other red flags[16,17] that can alert the surgeon to issues that increase the likelihood of complications of any kind, especially unhappiness or dissatisfaction (**Box 1**).[18]

Expectations

During the consultation this aspect should be discussed in great detail one or more times as necessary with the patient. Expectations are divided in two areas: procedural and surgical.

Procedural

A general overview of the surgery experience during consultation is helpful to orient the patient as to how their day will go and what they will likely experience. Give them a few names of patients who have had surgery at the clinic and who are willing to share their experience. Also, a preoperative telephone call or visit to go over specific details of the surgical day is important to ensure protocol is followed (**Box 2**).

Surgical

This aspect is very important and must be discussed in detail with the patient verbally and in writing (patient consent form) during the consultation and before the surgery (**Box 3**).

Blood Supply of the Scalp

Adequate blood supply of the scalp is critical for the success of HTS and a comprehensive preoperative evaluation should be done, including previous scars, smoking status, previous hair transplants, and scarring alopecias. The scalp is a unique and well-vascularized structure receiving blood flow from five major paired arteries: (1) supratrochlear, (2) supraorbital, (3) temporal, (4) posterior auricular, and (5) occipital. The circulation comes from the periphery to the center, where there are many anastomoses (**Fig. 3**). There are no significant perforants and most of the area receives a direct cutaneous supply. Any damage to the main supply may impact the circulation of the scalp in

the center especially with those patients with hair loss and previous scars after trauma, burns, scarring alopecia (lichen plano pilaris, pseudopelade of Brocq, lupus) and postradiotherapy. Smokers and patients with previous hair transplant or scalp reductions may also have decreased blood circulation of the scalp. Knowledge of the scalp's vascular anatomy can lead to more effective HRS,[19] great hair growth and survival, and fewer complications. To avoid a complication, one should decrease epinephrine concentration in the tumescent solution and avoid dense packing technique, planting no more than 25 to 35 grafts/cm^2. It is important to evaluate the blood supply of the scalp in both donor and recipient areas, looking for any signs of ischemia during the surgery and during the postoperative period.

Intraoperative

This section discusses the most common intraoperative complications.

Box 1
Red flags during the consultation

1. Body dysmorphic disorder
2. Patients with great expectations
3. The rude or pushy patient (narcissistic personality)
4. The indecisive or vague patient (passive-aggressive personality)
5. The perfectionist (obsessive-compulsive personality)
6. The shopper
7. The plastic or hair (surgiholic)
8. The patient with minimal deformity (body dysmorphic disorder)
9. The patient who praises the surgeon excessively and denigrates colleagues (borderline personality disorder)
10. The patient with psychologic or psychiatric issues (bipolar, schizophrenic)
11. The "very important patient" (classic narcissistic personality)
12. The patient with recent loss (depression)
13. The patient who does not wish to be photographed
14. The patient who hides the fact that they are under some type of treatment
15. The patient who makes the surgeon's office his or her home
16. The immature patient
17. Familial disapproval
18. The secretive patient (absolute secrecy about the surgery)
19. The patient unsatisfied or unhappy with previous HRS

Bleeding

During HTS bleeding rarely if ever is sufficient to cause serious problems. Because the surgery is performed in the upper reaches of the subcutaneous layer of the scalp, bleeding comes from capillaries and arterioles (subdermal plexus) and can usually be managed with the use of dilute epinephrine in a tumescent solution or in the local anesthetic or even by simply applying pressure. Tumescence of the donor and recipient scalp elevates the follicles above the deep subcutaneous arteriolar plexus, minimizing bleeding during follicular harvesting and when creating recipient site incisions (**Fig. 4**).

HTS is an elective surgery and may not be performed on patients currently taking anticoagulant medications (Coumadin, heparin, Plavix) for various medical conditions or on patients with high blood pressure, diabetes, and so forth until a preoperative medical clearance and drug management is obtained and coordinated with the appropriate medical specialist. Other substances with antiplatelet activity, such as aspirin, nonsteroidal anti-inflammatory drugs, vitamin E, and alcohol, also should be stopped 1 week before surgery to reduce the risk of excessive intraoperative or postoperative bleeding. Herbal supplements (side effect blood thinners), such as Gingko biloba, chromium picolinate, and ginseng, should also be discontinued for 2 weeks before the surgery.

If the tumescence solution and depth level of the donor harvesting is done properly there should be no disruption of important arteries and veins. If bleeding of the donor area occurs it is important to apply pressure in the area and look for the source; after the source of bleeding is found, one can continue to apply pressure (capillaries) until a clot is formed or gently use a hemostat (bigger vessels). Some surgeons coagulate the vessels using electrocautery for homeostasis, but the authors recommend a ligature with absorbable suture. It is important to evaluate patients for hematoma detection and treatment during the surgery and in the postoperative period. Excessive scalp bleeding in the recipient area can obscure the operative field and interfere with the insertion of grafts into the recipient sites. The result is often traumatized grafts and prolonged operative times, which ultimately decrease follicular unit survival. It is critical to evaluate and reinforce the anesthetic-vasoconstrictor effect of the scalp before and

---

Box 2
Procedural expectations

1. Time to report to the surgery center, give directions, map, telephone numbers
2. What laboratory studies will be done (if applies)
3. Any medical clearance completed (if applies)
4. No blood thinners for 3 to 5 days before surgery; some specific cases require an approval from the specialist and surgeon
5. Discontinue herbal supplements for 2 weeks before surgery
6. No exercise or alcohol for 5 days before surgery
7. Wear a button-down shirt on the day of surgery
8. Wash the hair the night before and the morning of the day of surgery
9. Length of the surgery
10. Most patients receive premedication (Valium or Versed) and need a ride to and from the surgery center
11. Patient may come to the office the morning after surgery for evaluation and hair shampoo
12. How long the patient will be out of work
13. Cost; it is critical in plastic surgery and HTS to cover the financial matters before surgery, and fees should be paid in advance

---

Box 3
Surgical

1. Premedication given before the surgery
2. Type of anesthesia
3. Painless to light discomfort during the application of the local anesthetic during and after the surgery
4. Surgical plan; patient concerns should be discussed
5. Edema, bleeding
6. Visits to the office including suture removal and follow-ups
7. Scarring in the donor area
8. What to expect after the surgery the first 10 days, and 4, 8, and 12 or more months, including unsynchronized growth of the transplanted hair
9. Medical clearance is necessary for those patients with diabetes, high blood pressure, heart problems, and so forth, including medications before, during, and after surgery. The surgeon and patient should be aware of any recommendations of the specialist
10. Naturalness with hairline asymmetry; irregular pattern should be expected
11. Photography is critical in plastic and HTS; preoperative pictures always must be taken and compared with postoperative pictures

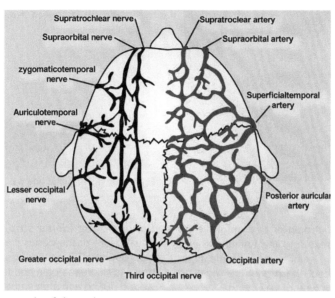

Fig. 3. Blood and nerve supply of the scalp.

during the creation of the recipient site and placing stages. Inadequate local anesthesia means the vasoconstrictive effect of epinephrine is suboptimal and more bleeding ensures. Patient discomfort (stiff neck, sore back, even a full bladder) can contribute to additional scalp bleeding. Good preoperative screening and patient education and guidance during the procedure minimize or prevent most of the problems associated with excess scalp bleeding during HTS.

Pain control

With the new medications and techniques at the surgeon's disposal, HRS should be relatively painless. Generally speaking, premedication using oral Valium or intravenous Versed is given to most patients before starting the surgery. This helps to reduce patient anxiety, pain, or discomfort during the local anesthetic infiltration and even produces a mild amnesic effect.

For those cases when the premedication is not given, the use of topical anesthetic (LMX-4, lidocaine 4%) reduces pain during anesthetic infiltration.[20] A ring block is best for this procedure using a 50:50 mixture of 1% lidocaine and 0.25% marcaine. Tumescent solution (saline solution plus epinephrine, 1:100,000–400,000) for vasoconstriction is then used to augment the ring block and protect the vascular bed in the lower subcutaneous scalp minimizing scalp bleeding. Scalp tumescence facilities graft placement by reducing bleeding and increasing the space between the follicular units. Prevention is important, and several times during the surgery the patient

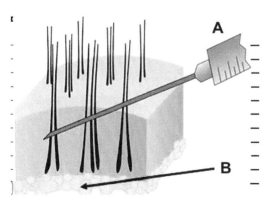

Fig. 4. Tumescence solution, two planes. (A) Intradermal and (B) subcutaneous.

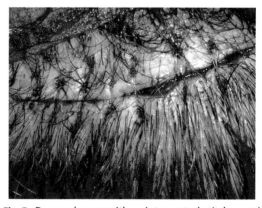

Fig. 5. Donor closure with uninterrupted stitches and small gaps.

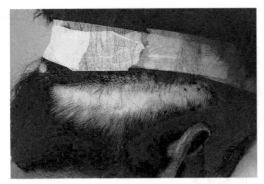

Fig. 6. Wide scar.

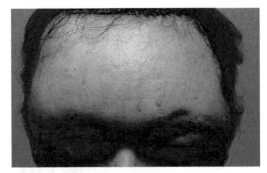

Fig. 7. Day 4 PO, facial edema.

should be asked about pain or discomfort in the donor or recipient areas and the anesthetic and tumescent solution reinforced. Medications administered throughout the procedure must be documented on some type of flow chart.

In some hair restoration practices supraorbital and supratrochlear nerve block are also used to augment the ring block.[21] Before the surgery is finished it is also recommended to administer a local infiltration of Marcaine 0.25% in the donor area to minimize pain or discomfort in the 4 to 6 hours following the surgery. Ketoprofen, 30 to 60 mg intramuscularly, can also be administered at the end of the surgery to minimize postoperative pain.

Box 4
HTS side effects

1. Bleeding: +
2. Pain: +−++
3. Edema: +−++
4. Tightness in the donor area: +−++
5. Ingrown hair: weeks to months following HTS
6. Cyst formation: weeks to months following HTS
7. Numbness of the scalp: 6–12 or more months.
8. Temporary loss (shock loss) of the nontransplanted hair: anagen or telogen effluvium +−++. Regrowth is expected in weeks to months.
9. Temporary loss of the transplanted hair: +−++++: anagen or telogen effluvium. Regrowth is expected in weeks or months.
10. Itching of the scalp: +
11. Dry scalp: +
12. Hiccups: +

Side effect: + and ++.
Complication: +++−++++ (except #9).
Data from Perez-Meza D. Complications in HRS. In: Programs and abstracts. IX Orlando Live Surgery workshop, 2003.

Donor closure (donor strip)

The closure of the donor area is a very important step during HTS. Several issues should be monitored to decrease pain and tightness of the donor wound during and after surgery. The objective is to produce the least visible scar while preserving the integrity of the donor scalp vascularity.[22]

Wound tension should be minimal or absent for an optimal donor scar. Care should be taken to assess the elasticity of the scalp when planning the dimensions of a donor strip. With today's large grafting sessions, more donor tissue is required to obtain the surgical goals (number of grafts). Wider (1.5–2 cm) and longer (>30 cm) donor strips are harvested for this reason. The Mayer-Pauls Scalp Elasticity scale measures the laxity of the donor scalp and for each value recommends a corresponding maximum strip width.[23] This scale is a guide for the estimation of the donor area that can be safely closed with minimal tension. Generally speaking, the tighter a scalp feels, the longer and narrower the donor strip should be with a maximum width of about 10 to 15 mm for best results, but this varies for each patient. Care should be taken to minimize donor strip width around the mastoid process because the scalp is always tighter and thinner in this area. If there is tension when approximating the wound edges,

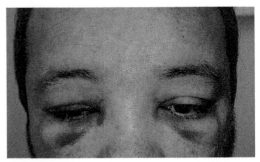

Fig. 8. Day 7 PO, bilateral palpebral edema and bruising.

undermining of the wound edges 0.5 to 1 cm in the deep subcutaneous layer (above the galea if it is present) can greatly reduce the tension of the wound closure. The use of a single or multilayer closure technique with sutures or staples seems to have a bearing on the quality of the scar produced including those cases with hyperelasticity of the scalp, such as Ehlers-Danlos syndrome, where a two-layer closure is always recommended. The number of layers used also depends on whether or not the patient has had prior surgeries (decreases scalp elasticity); the width of the donor strip; and the surgeon's preference.

If there is too much tension in the donor area to reapproximate the wound edges safely, the area should be packed with moist gauze and left alone for 1 to 3 hours until all the tumescent and anesthetic solutions have been reabsorbed. Towel clamps can also be used to create a mechanical creep to stretch the scalp. If the wound cannot be closed after these measures, it is recommended to place interrupted stitches without tightening them completely, leaving small gaps between the wound edges (**Fig. 5**). Too much tension in the closure can produce ischemia, necrosis, or wound dehiscence (see **Fig. 1**) of the upper or lower flaps resulting in a wide scar and loss of donor hair (**Fig. 6**). If the closure is done with moderate to high tension, the patient should be informed of this and be given strong medication for pain and discomfort.

It should also be noted that patients of African descent have more tendency toward pathologic scars in the donor area versus whites, Hispanics, or Asians. With each subsequent HTS it is recommended to remove any previous scars when possible, minimizing the total visible scar. Prevention is important and it is recommended to remove

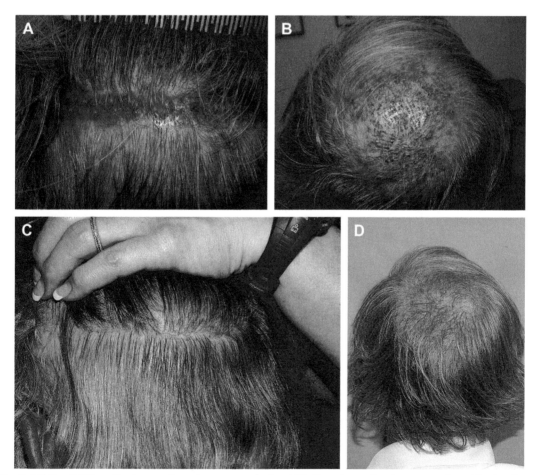

Fig. 9. (*A*) Day 7 PO, patient came for suture removal after HTS. Pustules and redness were found in the donor area. Culture was done and was positive for methicillin-resistant *Staphylococcus aureus*. Treatment consisted of oral doxycycline, oral Bactrim, and topical Bactroban cream. The patient responded quickly. (*B*) Day 7, recipient area also showing pustules. (*C*) At 8 months PO, donor area healed without complications. (*D*) Recipient area healed. (*Courtesy of* William Parsley, MD, Louisville, KY.)

a donor strip with minimum to no tension in the donor closure.

Difficult graft placement

Difficult graft placement can make a routine HTS last hours longer than expected. A number of factors can contribute to this complication. Anything that increases lateral pressure on a graft causes it to "pop" up when attempting to place another follicle in an adjacent site. Tissue edema resulting from numerous injections, traumatic graft placement, hypertension, excessive bleeding, and poor anesthesia all result in a worsening spiral of progressive edema and graft popping. The best way to control this is to manage anesthesia, blood pressure, and so forth in the early phase of surgery. Also, by placing grafts from the back to front of the scalp, tension is reduced minimizing further popping. Use of buddy placing technique (stick and place, whereby the surgeon makes the site and the technician places the graft) is also helpful under these circumstances.

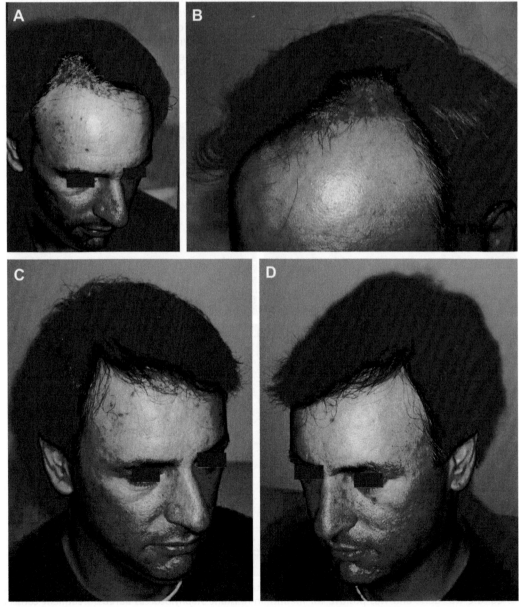

Fig. 10. Day 9 PO following HTS. Infection was noticed in the right recipient area (*A*) and left recipient area (*B*). (*C, D*) PO 12 months later both areas healed without complication. (*Courtesy of* Antonio Ruston, MD, Sao Paulo, Brazil.)

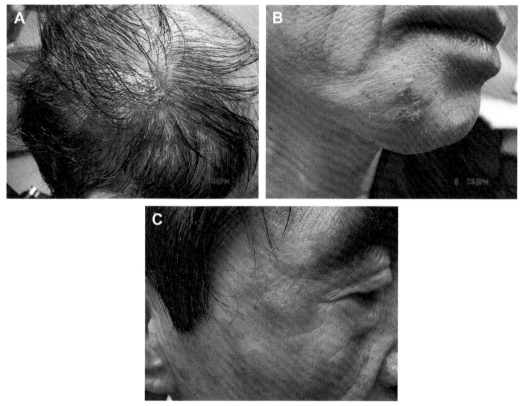

Fig. 11. (A–C) Herpes zoster case.

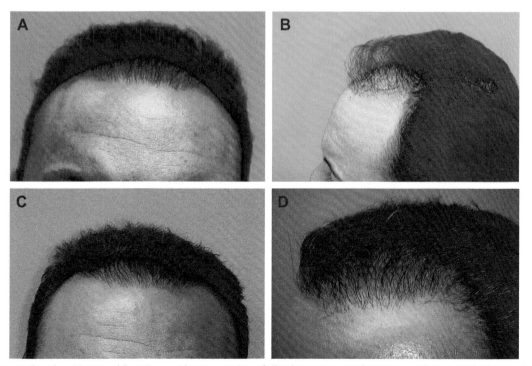

Fig. 12. (A, B) A 39-year-old patient with one previous follicular unit transplantation, unhappy with the results (pluggyness and hairline design). He also lost more hair in the mid-scalp. (C, D). One year follow-up after corrective surgery (1200 grafts) and medical treatment.

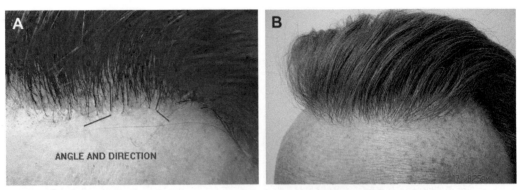

Fig. 13. (*A*) Before view of a 45-year-old patient with two previous HTS. Note unnatural hairline with pitting and pluggyness including wrong angle and direction. (*B*) At 1 year PO after one corrective surgery with follicular unit transplantation.

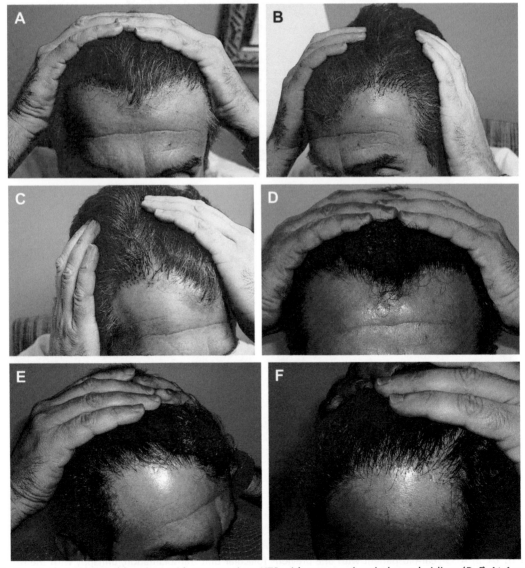

Fig. 14. (*A–C*) A 38-year-old patient with two previous HTS with unnatural and pluggy hairline. (*D–F*) At 1 year after three restoration surgeries: punch excision (removing the old plugs and suture) and recycling of the grafts and follicular unit transplantation.

Graft-recipient site mismatch is another source of difficult graft placement. If the size of the graft is either too big or too small for the intended recipient site, the graft implantation phase of the surgery can be extremely difficult. Struggling through a case this way ultimately leads to fatigue, frustration, and a poor result. It is vital to monitor the graft production process closely for consistency in graft size and shape. Likewise, making sure the recipient sites are a good fit for these follicles makes the entire surgery proceed much smoother. Check a sampling of grafts for ease of placement into a few test sites to avoid this pitfall.

Monitoring the graft production for consistency of size and shape reduces the likelihood that the recipient sites are not a good fit. Sometimes the surgeon also needs to adjust the size of the sites. In addition, gentle handling of the hair grafts, the use of good lightning and magnification (loupes), and continuous hydration of grafts all contribute to an easier implantation process.

Adverse reactions to medications or the operating room and office environment often go undetected. Patients may experience altered states of consciousness, becoming obtunded or agitated. HTS is unique in that the physician may not be in

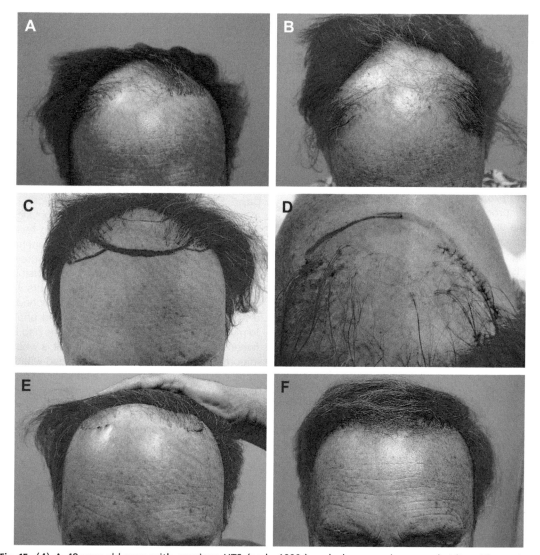

Fig. 15. (*A*) A 48-year-old man with previous HTS (early 1990s) and pluggy and uneven hairline. The patient wanted to remove the old plugs and conservative hair restoration of the hairline, front and mid-scalp. (*B*) Superior frontal view. (*C*) Surgical plan (first step) bilateral forehead lift for removing the hair plugs. (*D*) Immediate PO picture. (*E*) At 10 days PO. (*F*) At 6 months PO after second step; follicular unit transplantation (1400 grafts). (*Courtesy of* Ricardo Mejia, MD, Jupiter, FL and David Perez-Meza, MD, Maitland, FL.)

the operating room with the patient for periods of time during the surgery, usually during the graft implantation phase. Familiarization among surgeon and staff with the signs and symptoms of syncope, lidocaine toxicity, epinephrine overdose, drug interactions (β-blocker and epinephrine), allergic reactions, and an evolving cardiovascular event, such as a stroke or myocardial infarction, is critical to the patient's safety. Periodic review of emergency situations with operating room staff decreases the odds that a significant patient event is not overlooked. It is also important that the surgeon and lead nurse be advanced cardiac life support certified, have an algorithm ready in the operating room, periodically check the expiration date of all medications of the emergency kit, and have an automatic external defibrillator available. Prevention is the key. If a life-threatening situation occurs, stop the surgery, treat the patient immediately, and if necessary call 911 and transport the patient to the hospital for continuing treatment. The hair grafts can be preserved in saline solution or Custodiol solution in the refrigerator at 4°C until the HTS can be continued. Medical clearance is very valuable for those patients with certain preexisting conditions (high blood pressure, diabetes, coronary artery disease, and so forth).

Other problems

Other problems that can occur are directly related to the prolonged chair time (4–10 or more hours) often endured by patients undergoing so-called "mega" or "giga" sessions (2500–4000 or more grafts). Without an IV in place the risk of dehydration and hypoglycemia are significant unless proactive measures are taken throughout the duration of the procedure. The patient should have breakfast in the morning of the day of surgery. It is also important to give fluid and food to the patient during surgery. Deep venous thrombosis is also a significant risk for some patients. Encourage them to get up, stretch (neck, back, and legs), and walk about at prescribed intervals to decrease venous stasis.

Prolonged ischemia of the scalp after the grafts are planted may also delay appropriate wound healing and revascularization of the hair grafts and also may impact the hair growth and survival.[24]

Postoperative

This period starts as soon as the surgery is done and the patient leaves the surgery center. The postoperative instructions should be reviewed in detail with the patient or a family member; answering any questions is the best way to avoid any type of confusion or misunderstanding that can lead to

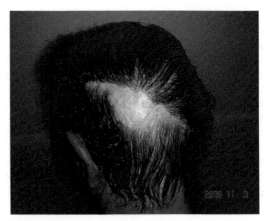

Fig. 16. Wide scar and hair loss in the donor area. (*Courtesy of* Antonio Ruston, MD, Sao Paulo, Brazil.)

a complication. For those patients whose primary language is not the same as the person giving the instructions, use an interpreter to avoid any miscommunication. The patient should have the surgeon's and nurse's telephone numbers available as a primary and secondary contact should they have any problems. A follow-up telephone call by the surgeon or a designated staff member to check on their well-being is always appreciated by the patient on the first or second postoperative day. Periodic postoperative evaluations at 4-month intervals allow the patient and physician to check their progress and a chance to review any questions and concerns. Give the patient honest feedback on the progress of their hair growth and make sure to plan their next follow-up visit before they leave the office. For those patients who live too far away to return to the office, schedule a telephone follow-up. Ask them to send photos to review whenever possible. Bridging the gap between the procedure and the end result is what is important. It keeps the surgeon engaged with the patient in a dialog facilitating the handling of problems both big and small. This period lasts from day

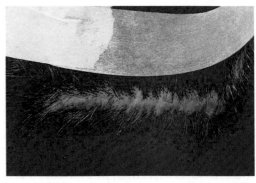

Fig. 17. Keloid scar in the donor area after two HTS.

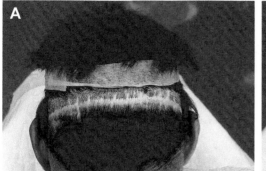
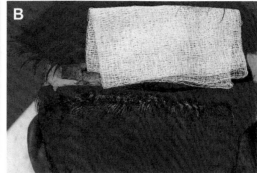

Fig. 18. (*A*) Before, hypertrophic scar in the donor area. (*B*) After, following donor harvesting including scar removal.

1 postoperative until 12 to 15 or more months after full hair regrowth is expected.

In the course of the preoperative conversation with the patient, it is important to distinguish between side effects and complications following HTS (**Box 4**.) In general, side effects, such as edema, are normal following surgery and should not be treated as a complication. Discussing edema as a normal part of the surgical recovery redefines it as something to be expected and not an unwanted surprise (ie, complication). Remember to discuss these issues before surgery.

Following HTS, the early postoperative period may be characterized by one of the following forms. First, it may be pleasant and painless. This usually happens with patients who have a normal personality, realistic expectations, and satisfactory interpersonal relationships. Second, psychologic disturbances may occur. Anxiety is common and sometimes depression is also found. These patients depend on others for reassurance about the wisdom of their decision to undergo this procedure and the eventual outcome of the surgery. The third form concerns the critical and

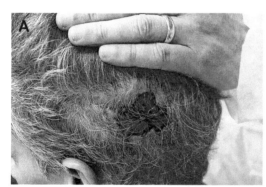
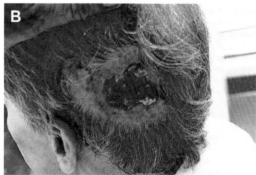
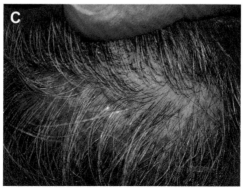

Fig. 19. (*A–C*) Necrosis in the donor area.

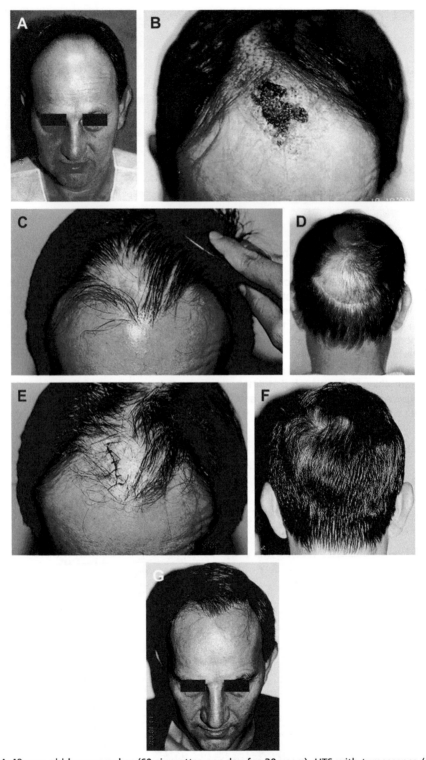

Fig. 20. (*A*) A 49-year-old heavy smoker (60 cigarettes per day for 20 years). HTS with tumescence (epinephrine 1:500,000), no dense packing in the recipient area. (*B*) At 3 days PO, first signs of ischemia, and 7 days PO a necrotic area in the central frontal area is observed. (*C*) Recipient area was kept clean with gentle cleansing and topical fibrinolitic once a day. Scar and hair loss after the area healed. (*D*) At 2 weeks PO, hair loss above the donor scar. Treatment with topical minoxidil 5% once a day. (*E*) Surgical excision of the scar. (*F*) Donor area, 8 months PO showing normal regrowth. (*G*) Recipient area 6 months PO after the excision showing good regrowth. (*Courtesy of* Antonio Ruston, MD, Sao Paulo, Brazil.)

demanding patient. The attitudes of the surgeon and the staff are the most important. A confident, firm, and encouraging attitude expressed frequently by the surgeon and staff is essential. Consistent and attentive postoperative care is also important to the outcome of the surgery. Anything that affects the postoperative period may cause, or lead to, a complication.

Following HTS, the course of the postoperative period is directly related to the wound healing process and revascularization of the hair transplant grafts.[24] It is critical to discuss with the patient when to expect preliminary and full results following the first, second, or more surgeries. It is very helpful to break this down into intervals commonly associated with visual or physical changes in their

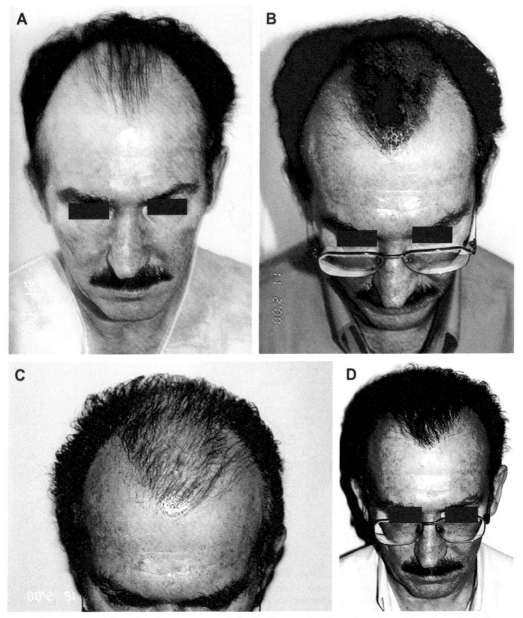

Fig. 21. (*A*) A 52-year-old smoker (20 cigarettes daily for 25 years). Discontinued smoking 2 weeks before and 2 weeks after the surgery. Tumescence solution in the recipient area (epinephrine 1:500,000). (*B*) At day 3 PO, necrotic area (2 cm × 5 cm) in the center of the scalp. Topical fibrinolitic and washing once a day. Donor area without complications. (*C*) One month PO, crust felt off spontaneously without hair regrowth. (*D*) Good regrowth after 8 months. (*Courtesy of* Antonio Ruston, MD, Sao Paulo, Brazil.)

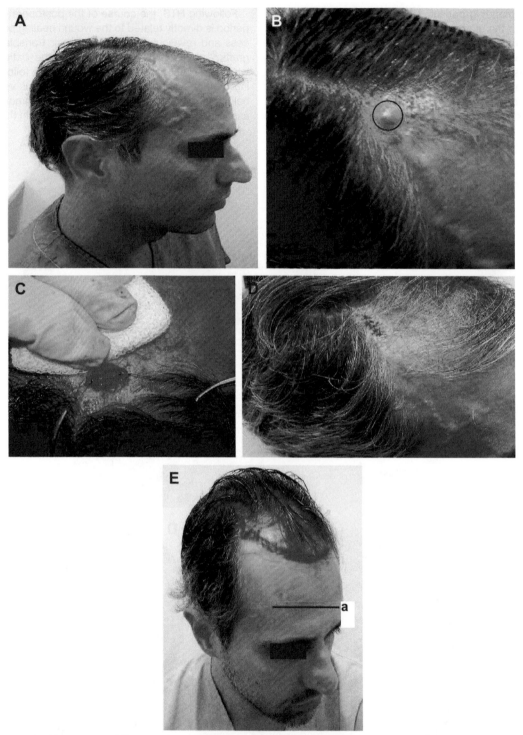

Fig. 22. (*A, B*) A 44-year-old man with Norwood Class 4. First HTS, with 1050 grafts in the hairline and front. At 2 weeks PO a pulsatil vein with swelling was found in the right side of the face. Clinical examination led to a diagnosis of fistula A-V. (*C*) A vascular surgeon performed a surgical ligation of the frontal vein. (*D*) Immediate PO. (*E*) A small swelling of the vein (*arrow*) is noticed in the preoperative picture. No evidence of recurrence was found. (*Courtesy of* Nicolas Lusicic, MD, and Alejandra Susacasa, MD, Buenos Aires, Argentina.)

scalp, including what occurs the first 3, 6, or more months after the procedure. Final results may be expected after 12 to 15 or more months following the procedure. Pictures are very important for evaluating progress and should be taken before the surgery and at each follow-up.

Bleeding

During the postoperative period bleeding can occur in either the donor or recipient areas. The patient leaves the office with a head band with gauze in the donor area and light pressure. If the patient notices a red spot on the bandage, this can be controlled by applying steady pressure with gauze over the bleeding area for 10 to 15 minutes. If the bleeding continues the patient should contact the office.

Patients are advised to come back the morning after surgery for evaluation of the donor and recipient areas and for a hair shampoo. The head band is removed and the donor site is evaluated for possible bleeding. Donor wound bleeding in the first few days after surgery needs to be checked for signs of an active arterial source or hematoma formation. Bright red color and persistent flow that do not respond to pressure dressings for a few hours,

and marked swelling suggesting a hematoma are sure signs that the wound should be explored and the source of bleeding identified. Make accommodations to evaluate the patient as soon as possible. Fortunately this is an uncommon postoperative event if the following steps are taken in the donor harvesting portion of the surgery. As previously mentioned, use a tumescent solution with epinephrine. Make sure to use an adequate amount to elevate the follicles above the deeper vascular structures and then wait 10 to 15 minutes for the vasoconstriction to ensue before excision of any tissue. Keep the plane of dissection just below the follicular bulbs in the subcutaneous fat and take care to avoid the larger occipital and posterior auricular vessels. Any bleeding from the donor wound that occurs after day 3 to 4 is most likely from a dissolving hematoma and evacuates itself without disrupting the closure. The patient should follow the indications to avoid any physical activity or work or discontinue any medication for high blood pressure, which may increase blood pressure and produce some type of bleeding.

The recipient site is treated the same as the donor site, and should also be evaluated for possible bleeding. Postoperative bleeding is usually the

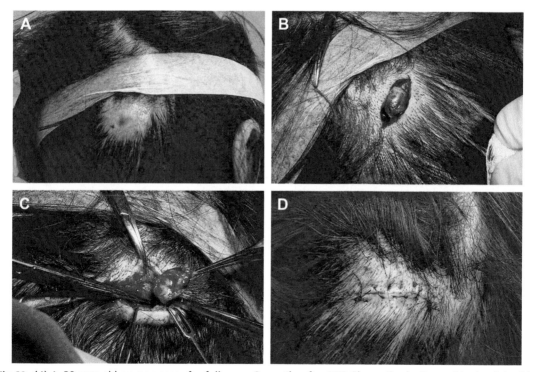

Fig. 23. (*A*) A. 38-year-old woman came for follow-up 2 months after HTS. She noticed a "tumor" in the right side of the donor area (scar) of the occipital area. The patient was evaluated and a pseudoaneurysm was found. There were no previous signs of bleeding. (*B, C*) Surgical excision was performed with 1.5-cm incision to localize the afferent artery that was ligated. The tumor was also removed. (*D*) Immediate PO. The patient was seen 6 months later with the area healed and no recurrence of the vascular lesion. (*Courtesy of* Matt Leavitt, DO, and David Perez-Meza, MD, Maitland, Florida.)

result of inadvertent trauma to the scalp causing the extrusion of one or a number of grafts. A prolonged anesthesia in the grafted area is common because the surface network of sensory nerves has been disrupted by the recipient site incisions. The loss of sensory input renders the patient's head movements a bit uncoordinated (ie, when getting in and out of a car). Making the patient aware of this phenomenon can help them make a conscious effort when moving around their environment for the first week. After this period the grafts are sufficiently stable to withstand mild trauma without extrusion. Patients should be discouraged from attempting to replace extruded

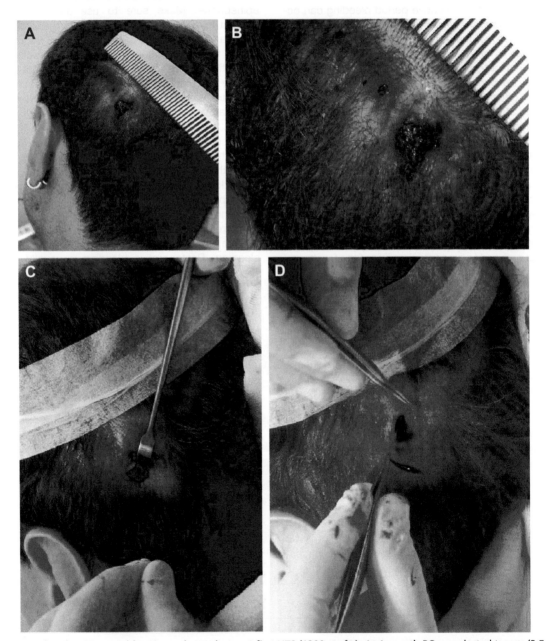

Fig. 24. (*A, B*) A 37-year-old patient who underwent first HTS (1200 grafts). At 1 month PO, a pulsated tumor (2.5 cm) was found in the donor area (left occipital). The tumor did not disappear and bled once. The patient was evaluated by a vascular surgeon and pseudoaneurysm was detected. (*C, D*) Surgical approach consisted of a 1-cm incision below the tumor to localize the afferent artery, which was ligated. The tumor was also excised and wounds closed. (*E*) Immediately PO. (*F*) At 5 months PO, areas healed and no recurrence. (*Courtesy of* Nicolas Lusicic, MD, and Alejandra Susacasa, MD, Buenos Aires, Argentina.)

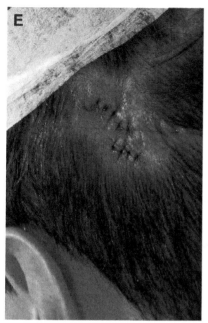 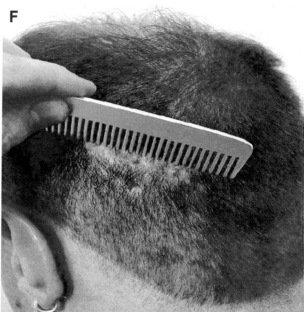

Fig. 24. (*continued*)

follicles because this usually leads to the displacement of additional grafts and they are not likely to survive anyway.

Some ethnics groups, such as Asians and Hispanics, have tendency to bleed more; this could be related to the fact that the hair follicles are deep (5 mm or more long). Here the tumescent effect is very valuable.

Edema

Edema occurs to a degree in every patient undergoing HTS, because this is a natural response to the trauma of surgery. Minimal edema should be expected during the 4 days postoperative. Strictly speaking, this is not considered a true complication but rather it is a surgery side effect (see **Box 4**), but when the swelling is extensive enough to cause visual obstruction and pain from accumulation in the eyelids and periorbital areas (**Figs. 7** and **8**) it qualifies as a complication, especially when certain measures can be taken to minimize the likelihood of this phenomenon. Many hair transplant surgeons advocate the use of a tumescent solution infused with steroids (triamcinolone) injected into the recipient areas[25,26] with or without postoperative oral steroids (Medrol dose pack or oral prednisone) to reduce significantly the risk of serious postoperative facial edema. In addition, it is important to make sure the patient understands the value of decreased physical activity,[27] especially forward bending of the head. It is recommended to recline intermittently with ice packs on the forehead during

the first 3 postoperative days. Because the movement of the fluid is primarily driven by gravity, patients should be taught how to use this to their advantage. There is some controversy regarding the real value of sleeping at a 45-degree angle during the first 3 days after surgery for reducing edema. Supine or lateral decubitus position without head elevation may prevent forehead edema.[28] Minimal edema in the donor area is expected.

Pain

The patient should expect minimal to no pain or minimal discomfort in the donor and recipient areas. Most of the time, Tylenol as needed is sufficient; some patients may need stronger medication for pain. Light tightness of the donor area can also be expected during the first days following surgery; laser therapy also helps to reduce the tightness.[29] If the patient has severe pain, discomfort, and tightness in the donor area Percocet or Tradol are recommended. Sometimes a pillow produces some pressure in the sutured areas; the patient should rest and sleep on one of the sides (temporal areas).

Infection

The scalp is a very well-vascularized area and an infection in the donor or recipient areas is an uncommon event in HTS patients. The incidence has been reported as less than 0.1%, but most are anecdotal and usually caused by staphylococcus organisms. Although both gram-positive and gram-negative bacteria have been isolated, fungal infection could be another source of infection. Methicillin-resistant *Staphylococcus aureus* infection after HTS (**Figs. 9** and **10**), although rare, has been reported consistent with the increased frequency seen in outpatient facilities or especially with the occurrence of two surgery cases together (same day or same week).[30] Herpes zoster outbreak in the head and neck area following HTS has been reported (**Fig. 11**). In the United States and around the world some hair transplant offices often use antibiotic prophylaxis to reduce the risk of infection, despite the fact that studies have not supported this practice. There are many variables for the use of prophylactic antibiotics in HTS.[31] Usually an oral cephalosporin antibiotic is recommended, or clindamycin if the patient is allergic to penicillin. The dosage varies from only one dosage of 500 mg to 1 g, 1 hour before the surgery, and may be followed by 500 g postoperative twice a day for 5 days. Hair restoration patients with cardiac lesions require specific guidelines for endocarditis prophylaxis.[32] It is recommended that a medical clearance be obtained for appropriate treatment recommendations.

Prions (nonbacterial, nonviral protein pathogens without any DNA) have emerged as a new source of infections in surgery centers throughout Europe. Resistant to eradication by sterilization, prions have prompted the use of disposable surgical instruments in these regions. Prions have not been implicated as a source of infection in the United States.

Prevention of infection is important; some countries, such as the United Kingdom, have regulations including implementation of infection control policies.[33] There are also patient wound infection risk factors, such as age, nutritional status, diabetes mellitus, smoking, obesity, immunocompromised status, and infection at other body sites.

There are several measures to be followed for prevention and infection control: asking the patient to wash the hair the night before and in the morning of the surgery day; the operating room should be clean and decontaminated; sterilized material should be used; the surgeon and staff must use gloves, mask, gowns, and footwear covers for each patient and change gloves as necessary; hands should be properly washed; donor area asepsis with Hibiclens or Betadine after cutting the hair; the use of disposable instruments should follow as much as possible; the patient should have protective wear; and antibiotic prophylaxis (surgeon's personal preference). The HTS should be delayed or cancelled if the patient has an upper respiratory infection, gastrointestinal infection, uncontrolled diabetes, skin infection, or other type of infection that puts the patient in high risk of infection. Contagious diseases (hepatitis C, HIV-positive, Venereal Disease Research Laboratories–positive, and so forth) should also be evaluated properly.

Naturalness

With the new instrumentation and techniques, patients are expecting natural results following HTS. Hair loss is progressive and the surgeon and the patient should be aware of this; planning the hairline and surgical plan should include present and future hair loss, donor area availability, hair color and texture, age, budget, and so forth. Hairline location is very important in hair restoration, and there are several guidelines for its placement.[34,35] The surgeon should be very cautious in designing and surgical technique; hairline is the surgeon's signature. It is the unintended visual consequences of any or all of the following: an ill-conceived surgical plan, poor surgical technique, patient noncompliance, or an unexpected intraoperative event. Excluding the latter two circumstances (these are not really under the surgeon's control), good planning and proper technique can reduce the incidence and severity of aesthetic complications. Unnatural appearance of transplanted hair is a complication of a poor design and surgical execution (**Fig. 12**). With the advent of follicular unit hair transplantation, the surgeon should plan on recreating a pattern of hair growth that is seen in nature. A relatively low hairline does not look good if the patient has thin hair everywhere else. Creating zones of variable density in a patient with a Norwood V pattern to mimic the distribution pattern of hair in someone who is a Norwood III gives a very natural result. To transplant hair to suit the patient's desire without applying proper aesthetic principals is a breach of the physician's responsibility. If the hairline is low or pluggy or there is improper angulation of the hair grafts (**Figs. 13** and **14**), this is a complication. It is important to discuss with the patient that some times performing two or more HTS is required to resolve the problem and fix the complication. The treatment option varies from follicular unit transplantation or punch excision or recycling, forehead lift, or laser hair removal (**Fig. 15**).

Follicular single unit or multiunit transplantation is the gold standard in HRS but the right angle and the direction of the transplanted hair are critical to the outcome and naturalness following HRS, especially in the hairline and frontal areas. Also, placing one-hair follicular units in the first row and two-hair follicular units behind is the key for successful results; if the planning and surgical technique are not adequate it could result in a complication.

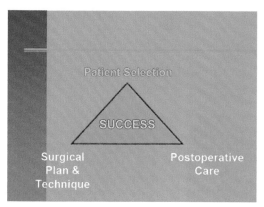

Fig. 25. Keys to success in HTS.

Prevention is related to designing a conservative hairline, especially with surgeons with little experience, and making the recipient sites in the right angle and direction. Some patients like the hairline restoration as it was 5 to 20 years before; the surgeon wisely should discuss with the patient all the pros and cons when designing the hairline. If the surgeon is not sure about hairline location, it is

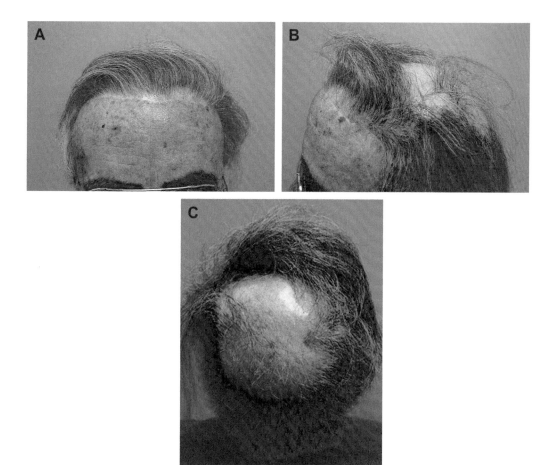

Fig. 26. (*A–C*) A 58-year-old patient with previous bilateral scalp surgery in the late 1980s. Several problems are shown: scar in the hair line, incorrect hair angle and direction, uneven hairline, baldness in the mid-scalp and crown areas, scars in the donor areas, and tight scalp. He came for evaluation, and his main concern was the hairline.

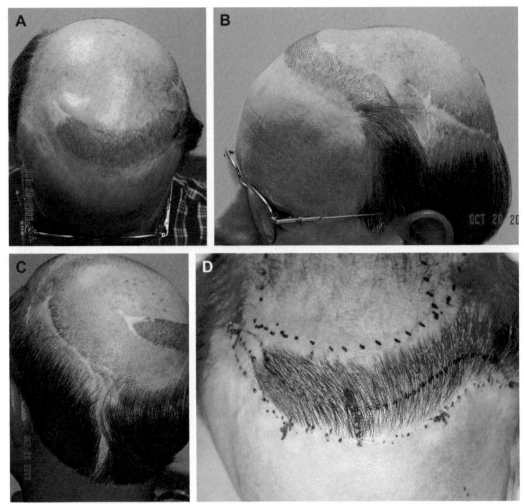

Fig. 27. Combining HST techniques. (*A–C*) A 45-year-old man with bilateral temporo-pariental-occipital (TPO) flaps 20 years previously and subsequent extensive hair loss now wears a hair piece. He wants to eliminate the hair system, correcting the flaps and eliminate the scarring. Several surgeries were performed over 8 months to correct the problem. (*D*) Stage 1 is a brow lift with excision of half anterior TPO flap and transplantation of excised hair in the anterior scalp. (*E*) Stage 2 is a flap advancement to excise the reminder of the anterior TPO flap, Z-transposition to correct the blunted temporal angle on the left, and transplantation of the excised hair in the themed scalp. Stage 3 is an extensive scalp lift with repair of the left TPO donor scar and excision of the posterior flap. HTS is performed with the excised hair in to the anterior scalp and hairline. Stage 4 is a standard HTS with grafts placed in to the crown. He had a total of 6500 follicular unit grafts. (*F–I*) Results after 15 months follow-up. (*Courtesy of* Robert Niedbalski, DO, and Antonio Mangubat, MD, Seattle, WA.)

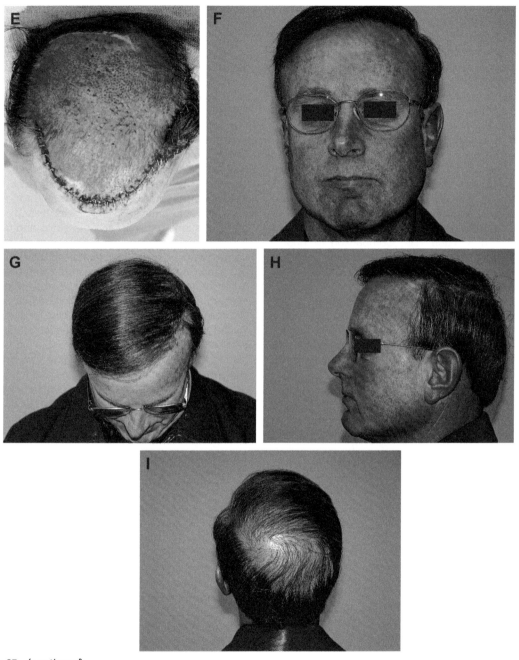

Fig. 27. (continued)

always safer and recommended to place it higher than lower. If the hairline is higher another surgery can be done to lower the hairline. If the hairline is low it is a complication and requires one or more surgeries to be fixed.

UNHAPPY AND UNSATISFIED PATIENT

Some unsatisfied or unhappy patients following HRS are reasonable people whose operations have not come out well and whose results are not up to either their expectations or those of the surgeon. The result is a surgical or psychologic complication. If it is a surgical complication, the medical-surgical treatment options should be evaluated. If plan A failed, one needs to be sure that plan B or C will work. The management of psychologic complication is part of the surgeon's job and all the aspects of the case should be revised including preoperative consultation, surgical plan, and surgical technique. Many patients are anxious to see the results in the first 3 to 6 months after the surgery, but keep in mind that the final results are seen in 12 or more months in most HTS cases. Follow-ups after the surgery are very important to evaluate the patient's progress. The photographic record is critical and pictures should be taken at each visit. Comparison of photographs, particularly with high resolution, can often be a great tool in demonstrating the amount of improvement that the surgery has produced. The use of the videomicroscope[36] with 50x power is also a valuable instrument. Many patients and their families quite honestly forget the appearance before the surgery. The best advice for the patients is to be patient and to wait to see the progress and final result.

Scarring: Keloid or Hyperthrophic

This is more likely to be a problem in the donor rather than the recipient area. With modern surgical techniques for donor harvesting and donor closure including the thricophytic technique,[2,37] scars have been improved dramatically and most of the time are unapparent or unnoticeable. With the advent of follicular unit grafting, recipient site incisions have become much smaller and shallower. The resultant scars heal much like a "paper cut" and are virtually undetectable. When significant scarring is seen after HTS, it is usually the result of poor planning or surgical technique in the removal of donor hair using the strip harvesting method (the most common technique for donor hair removal in contemporary HTS). Keloid or hypertrophy scars can be related to too munch tension in the suture line and the result of stretch (**Figs. 16** and **17**), wound dehiscence, or necrosis. With attention to the following basic principles, donor scars can be very inconspicuous, even when the hair is closely cropped.

Follicular transection should be avoided when excising the donor strip. Using a single scalpel blade to carve a free-hand donor ellipse produces much less follicular transection when compared with multibladed scalpels. Making an initial scoring incision through the dermis and then using countertraction on the wound edges and blunt

dissection in the subcutaneous layer can eliminate most of the follicular transection during the donor harvesting phase of surgery.

Donor strips taken from the portion of the occipital scalp without a separate galeal layer (the bottom 1–2 cm of hair-bearing scalp in the occipital area) tends to stretch significantly in the months following surgery. Keeping the donor excision at the level of the nuchal ridge eliminates this concern.

Remove old donor scars with each subsequent HTS whenever possible (**Fig. 18**). Note that any residual scar tissue below the surface reduces the elasticity of the scalp, so it is advisable to keep the donor strip width to 12 mm or less. If additional donor tissue is required, and the scalp and scar tissue allow, a secondary 2-mm or more strip can be removed once the extent of the subcutaneous scar tissue is known. If an active keloid scar is found in the donor area, there are several options: circular massage (improve circulation and reorient the collagen fibers) several times a day for several weeks; sessions of intralesional injection of triamcinolone; injection of 5-fluorouracil solution may also reduce the symptoms and scar size; and follicular unit extraction has also been used for scar grafting. Scar revision can be recommended but the patient should be aware that the resultant scar could be bigger than the first one.

Hair Growth and Survival, Multifactor Chain of Reaction, Poor Growth, the Silent Complication

Hair growth and survival of transplanted hair can be difficult to source. Generally speaking, a 92% to 95% hair growth and survival can be expected following HTS. A complication occurs when the production is below that percentage after 12 to 15 months postoperative. There are many factors that influence hair growth and survival.[38,39] Not to diminish the importance of good preoperative and postoperative care, but an in-depth analysis of the individual steps in the operating room from the harvesting of donor tissue, graft dissection, through the implantation phase of grafts usually reveals significant insights into the problem. That is because the hair follicle is most likely to be rendered unviable during this interval as a result of one or more of the following culprits.

Dehydration

Dehydration has been shown to cause poor growth more than any of the usual stressors typically encountered during HTS.[40] Follicles can be exposed to the air for prolonged periods during graft preparation, storage, and placement. Care should be taken to provide a moist environment during all phases of the procedure. A protocol should be established outlining the handling of tissue and be closely monitored for compliance. This complication can be prevented by keeping the grafts "hydrated" from the beginning to the end of the surgery.

Trauma

Trauma to grafts usually occurs during the implantation step. Inexperienced staff, irregular graft sizes, popping, and poorly designed recipient sites conspire to impose unnecessary trauma on the tissue to be transplanted. Taking the time regularly to inspect the grafts as they are being produced helps staff improve the consistency of graft size and shape necessary to produce recipient sites

that accommodate them. Overwhelming staff with recipient sites that are too densely packed or just too numerous for their skill level guarantees poor graft survival.

Out-of-body time

Out-of-body time for hair grafts has been demonstrated to have a negative impact on graft survival after 6 hours,[41] because more time decreases hair survival. Tissue preservation between the donor and recipient area is an important link that should lead to 100% survival. Normal saline has been the graft storage solution most often used in the past, but recent studies have shown improved graft survival within that 4- to 48-hour window when tissue is maintained in solutions enhanced

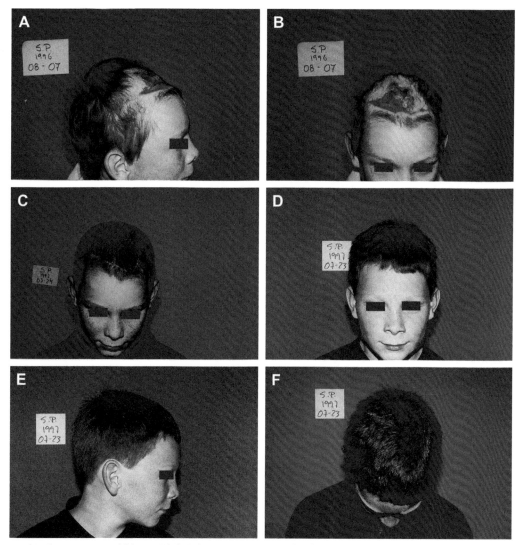

Fig. 28. (*A, B*) An 11-year-old boy with hair loss posttrauma in the frontoparietal area. (*C–F*) Views after skin flap prepared with the use of a 250-mL tissue expander. (*Courtesy of* Jerzy Kolasinski, MD, PhD, and Malgorzata Kolenda, MD, PhD, Poznan, Poland.)

with a variety of additives or "goodies" including antioxidants; Ph balance; electrolytes; amino acids; and membrane protection including prevention of intracellular swelling,[42] antiapoptotic effect, reduction of free radicals, and cytoprotective action including the autologous growth factors.[43] They provide several benefits for the grafts until they are placed back into the body. It is recommended to increase hair growth and survival by reducing the surgery time to 6 or less hours. More research is needed in this area.

Toxins

Toxins can be a source of poor growth if grafts are exposed during the course of HTS. Sterile water is lethal to hair grafts, as is Hibiclens (a common skin disinfectant used in many operating rooms). Try to eliminate any mistakes by removing any product from the operating room that is toxic to graft tissue and clearly marking all fluid containers (sterile water and saline for irrigation have similar containers).

Hydrogen peroxide

In most hair restoration practices, hydrogen peroxide is used in different dilutions (0.75%–1.5%) to remove blood during HTS. There is some controversy of positive (stimulates angiogenesis) and negative (delays wound healing and poor growth)

effects.[44] Until there is further research and information about the role of hydrogen peroxide, the exclusive use of saline solution during HTS is recommended.

Folliculitis

Folliculitis can be a cause of hair loss in the donor and recipient areas, as discussed previously.

Factor X

In 1984, it was postulated by Shiell[45] that in addition to the known causes of poor growth or follicular destruction, there was an unknown cause or "X factor," which may be responsible for loss of follicles. To date the cause of factor X has not been found and the search for the cause continues.

Factor H

One of the factors that may produce poor growth and poor hair quality can be related to trimming too much of the hair grafts before placing them in tiny recipient sites.[46–48] The surrounding tissue around the hair graft and papilla is important for hair growth, survival, and skeletonization (removing all the fat around the graft).

Dense packing does not mean dense growing; several studies have shown that increasing the grafts by centimeter squared may impact the hair

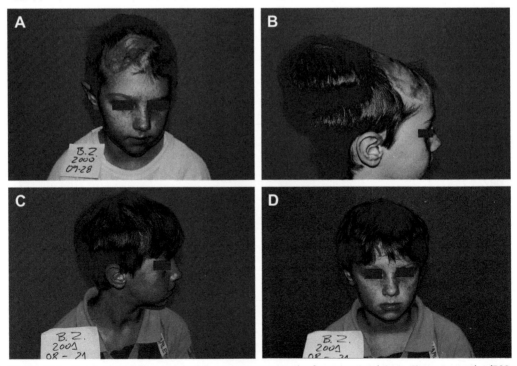

Fig. 29. (A, B) An 8-year-old patient with hair loss posttrauma in the frontoparietal Area. Tissue expander (500 mL) was used. (C–D) Views after scar correction with skin flaps and hair transplantation obtained from the dog-ears. (*Courtesy of* Jerzy Kolasinski, MD, PhD, and Malgorzata Kolenda, MD, PhD, Poznan, Poland.)

growth and survival. A total of 30 to 50 grafts cm^2 has shown 90% to 93% hair growth survival.[49,50] To date, there is no study to show great survival when planting 50 or more follicular units/cm^2. It is recommended to keep some fat around the hair grafts to increasing survival: chubby is better than skinny.

Inadequate blood supply of the scalp
Any factor that decreases the blood supply of the scalp may produce an ischemic and necrotic area in the donor and recipient area.

Donor area
The amount of epinephrine injected in the tumescent solution must be controlled during the HTS for all patients, but especially for those patients who have undergone one or more surgeries where the blood supply can be decreased. One should also be careful with smokers or diabetic patients. If too much vasoconstriction or too much tension for the donor closure is made, an ischemic and necrotic area can be produced. **Fig. 19**A shows a male patient 10 days postoperative after his third HTS. The donor area was closed with light to moderate tension. The patient came for suture removal and an area of necrosis (4 cm wide) in the left occipital area was found. Explaining the issue to the patient and giving him support was critical before starting treatment. Three weeks later the eschar has been separated spontaneously (**Fig. 19**B). The following is a summary of the treatment done:

1. Conservative management: No debridement of the necrotic tissue. If it is a partial-thickness necrosis area and debridement is performed, there is a high risk that a full-thickness wound can be produced. Let the necrotic area be localized and just cut the edges as necessary following the epitalization.
2. Wash the area twice a day.
3. Topical antibiotic and wound dressing twice a day.
4. Oral antibiotics are not recommended except if there is an infection; culture of the fluid if also indicated.
5. Follow-up every week. The eschar was separated spontaneously.
6. After 3 weeks the area healed and 5% Rogaine twice a day was recommended and low-level laser therapy.
7. The patient after 12 months. He had good regrowth (**Fig. 19**C).

In some cases, when there is full-thickness necrosis, conservative management should be done and the patient may need a skin graft or secondary closure if possible. A period of 6 months or more should pass before the patient is evaluated for secondary surgery.

Recipient area also can be susceptible to ischemia and necrosis. There are some possible causes related to the complication. Too much vasoconstrictor effect injected with the tumescent solution, especially in patients with previous hair transplant surgeries, previous scars after trauma or scarring alopecia, or dense packing technique. One must be careful how much vasoconstrictor is added.

Smokers

The risk of complications (poor healing, ischemia, and skin necrosis) for smokers who undergo plastic surgery from facelifts, abdominoplasty, and breast reductions[51–53] also has been mentioned in HTS.[54] Some of the effects of nicotine are vascular lesions from acute inflammation, occlusive thrombosis, and effects on microcirculation. Complications following hair transplant include ischemia, necrosis, and poor healing (**Figs. 20** and **21**).

It is recommended to stop smoking at least 2 to 3 weeks before and after the surgery. The following guidelines during the HTS are suggested: (1) decrease the amount of epinephrine in the tumescence solution, perhaps to 1:400,000 to 500,000; (2) place less than 25 to 30 grafts/cm^2; (3) avoid the dense packing technique; (4) close the donor area with minimum to no tension; and (5) monitor the patient during the postoperative period.

Arteriovenous Fistula and Aneurysm

These are rare complications that were more frequent with the old technique but can still be present following the modern HTS,[55,56] and the hair restoration surgeon should be aware of these complications and their treatment. Clinical examination and possible arteriogram help in the diagnosis. Prevention is important. If the fistula does not resolve spontaneously over a 3- to 6-month period, the surgical approach is recommended by ligating the afferent vein (**Fig. 22**). Pseudoaneurysm or aneurysms are also rare postoperative complications following HTS. The surgical approach (ligating the afferent vessel) is recommended (**Figs. 23** and **24**).

Summary

HTS has gained popularity because of natural results. As with any other surgical procedure a complication may occur. The complications can happen in the preoperative, intraoperative, and postoperative periods. The consultation is still a key part of the evaluation, especially related to patient expectations. Three factors are keys in a successful HTS: (1) patient selection, (2) adequate surgical plan and technique, and (3) postoperative care (**Fig. 25**).

SCALP SURGERY

Male and female pattern of hair loss are the most common forms of alopecia. There are also other causes, such as hormones, medications, postpartum, crash diet, anemia, trauma, burns, and so forth.

Scalp surgery was the initial surgical technique for the treatment of hair loss and scarring following trauma accidents and burns.[57] The use of scalp surgery for the treatment of avulsion of scalp was reported in 1911 by Davis.[57] He reviewed a series of 92 cases of scalping injury with treatment resulting in successful coverage in only 21 cases. In 1950, the avulsed scalp itself was used as split-thickness and full-thickness graft. In 1939, Okuda in Japan was the pioneer of the punch or hair plug technique to treat patients with hair loss. In 1959, Orentreich in New York reintroduced the technique.

During the 1960s to the early 1990s three surgical techniques were available to treat patients with hair loss in the scalp or other areas of the body caused by genetic, trauma, congenital, scarring, scalp infections, and so forth: (1) round and square punch technique (4 mm +);[58] (2) transplantation of donor strips of scalp hair;[59] and (3) transferal of local scalp flaps to the scalp,[60,61] eyebrows, or moustache. Also, free flaps and microsurgery were used for alopecia and avulsion of the scalp.[62] Each technique had pros and cons but complications were related to pluggyness, unnatural results, scarring in the donor and recipient areas, and unsatisfied patients. Alopecia reductions (removing bald tissue of the scalp) and scalp expansion had popularity.[63–69] Hair loss is progressive and many of those patients did not have medications available at that time to stabilize the hair loss following the scalp surgery, ending in a big area of baldness (**Fig. 26**).

The old punch technique was the state of the art from the late 1930s to the mid 1990s. Medicine advances everyday and with it the progress of surgical techniques including reduction of the hair graft size (from ≥ 4 mm to ≤ 1–2 mm); donor harvesting; graft preparation (microscope); and better instrumentation (tiny blades for the creation of the recipient sites). Follicular unit transplantation gained popularity in the mid 1990s; the results are natural with less complications or side effects versus the old punch technique and alopecia reductions. For all these reasons the popularity of scalp surgery or alopecia reductions has fallen to 1% to 2% or less of all the cases for the treatment of genetic hair loss. Also, the combination treatment with medical therapy (finasteride and minoxidil 2% and 5%) and low-level laser therapy has helped to stabilize hair loss and some type of regrowth.

Tissue expansion, tissue extension, scalp flaps, or follicular unit transplantation still play an important role for the treatment of hair loss after trauma, burns, congenital, and so forth for adults and children (**Figs. 27–29**).[70]

Nowadays, patients are seen who had some type of scalp surgery in the past and now they are looking to improve their results with corrective surgery. With the new surgical techniques moderate to great improvement can be done for those patients.

Summary

Scalp surgery for the treatment of male-pattern hair loss has decreased dramatically to less than 1% to 2% of all the HTS cases because of the natural results with modern follicular unit or multiunit transplantation. Tissue expansion, tissue extension, and flap rotation or advancement are still good surgical options for those patients with hair loss caused by trauma, burns, congenital, etc., and can be combined with HTS.

REFERENCES

1. Shapiro R. Follicular unit transplantation alone or follicular units with multigrafts: why, when, and how. In: Unger W, Shapiro R, editors. Hair transplantation. 4th edition. New York: Marcel Dekker, Inc; 2004. p. 435–68.
2. Unger W. How I use multi-follicular unit grafts. In: Unger W, Shapiro R, editors. Hair transplantation. 4th edition. New York: Marcel Dekker, Inc; 2004. p. 503–16.
3. Leavitt M. Hair loss in women. In: Programs and abstracts. 14th Annual Orlando Live Surgery Workshop. April 2008.
4. Bernstein R, Rassman W. The logic of follicular unit transplantation. Dermatol Clin 1999;17:277–96.
5. Cotterill P. President message. Hair Transplant Forum International 2007;7(2):42.
6. Perez-Meza D. Complications in hair restoration surgery. Hair Transplant Forum International 2000; 10(5):145.
7. Leavitt M. Corrective hair restoration. In: Stough D, Haber R, editors. Hair replacement. St. Louis: Mosby; 1996. p. 306–13.
8. Voguel JE. Correction of the cornrow hair transplant and other common problems in surgical hair restoration. Plast Reconstr Surg 2000;105(4):1528–36.
9. Unger W. Correction of cosmetic problems in hair transplanting. In: Unger W, Shapiro R, editors. Hair

transplantation. New York: Marcel Dekker; 2004. p. 663–87.

10. Perez-Meza D. Complications preoperative, intraoperative and post-operative following HTS. In: Programs and Abstracts. IX Annual Orlando Live Surgery Workshop; 2003.

11. Kaufman KD, Olsen EA, Whiting D. Finasteride in the treatment of men with androgenetic alopecia. J Am Acad Dermatol 1998;39:578–89.

12. Leavitt M, Perez-Meza D, Rao N, et al. Effects of finasteride 1 mg on hair transplant. Dermatol Surg 2005;(10):1268–76.

13. Olsen EA. A randomized clinical trial of 5% topical minoxidil vs 2% topical minoxidil and placebo in the treatment of AGA in men. J Am Acad Dermatol 2002;47(3):377–85.

14. Perez-Meza D. Low level laser therapy for the treatment of men with AGA. In: Programs and Abstracts of the 24th American Academy of Cosmetic Surgery meeting, Jan 2008. Orlando, Fl.

15. Goldwyn RM. Patient selection: importance of being cautious. In: Courtiss EH, editor. Aesthetic surgery: trouble-how to avoid it and how to treat it. St. Louis: Mosby; 1978.

16. Unger W. Body dysmorphic disorder. In: Unger W, Shapiro R, editors. Hair transplantation. New York: Marcel Dekker; 2004. p. 166–9.

17. Phillips KA. The broken mirror: understanding and treating body dysmorphic disorder. New York: Oxford University Press; 1996. [Revised and expanded edition 2005].

18. Musgrave R. Learning to say no. In: Kaye B, Gradinger G, editors. Symposium on problems and complications in aesthetic plastic surgery of the face. St. Louis: Mosby; 1984. p. 3–5.

19. Zuckerman J. Practical anatomic correlates to hair restoration surgery. International Journal of Aesthetic and Restorative Surgery 1995;3(2):93–4.

20. Perez-Meza D, Porcaro J. The use of topical anesthetic (LMX-4) for reducing pain and discomfort of the local anesthetic during hair transplant surgery. Poster Presentation. 14th Annual ISHRS meeting. San Diego, CA. Oct. 2006.

21. Seager D, Cam S. Supraorbital and supratrochlear nerve blocks in hair transplantation. In: Unger W, Shapiro R, editors. Hair transplantation. New York: Marcel Dekker; 2004. p. 255–8.

22. Mayer M, Perez- Meza D. Managing the donor area to minimize scarring. Int J Cosm Surgery and Aesthet Derm 2001;3:121–6.

23. Mayer M, Pauls T. Scalp elasticity scale. Hair Transplant Forum International 2005;15(4):122–3.

24. Perez-Meza D, Leavitt M, Mayer M. Growth factors part 1. Clinical and histological evaluation of the wound healing and revascularization of the hair graft after hair transplant surgery. Hair Transp Forum 2007;17(5):173–5.

25. Norwood O. Say goodbye to postoperative swelling. Hair Transplant Forum 1992;2(6):13.

26. Abassi G. Hair transplantation without post-operative edema. Hair Transplant Forum 2005;5(5):149,158.

27. Perez-Meza D. Postoperative instructions following hair transplant surgery. In: Programs and Abstracts of the 14th Orlando Live Surgery Workshop, April 2008.

28. Hwang S. Post-surgery: how to avoid facial swelling. In: Programs and Abstracts of the 14th Orlando Live Surgery Workshop, April 2008.

29. Andrews W, Perez-Meza D, Puig C. The use of laser therapy in the donor area following hair transplant surgery. In: Programs and Abstracts. 16th Annual ISHRS meeting, Las Vegas, Nevada. Sep 2007.

30. True R. Hair restoration in the age of MRSA. Hair Transplant Forum Int 2008;130–1, Pages 127.

31. Randall JK. Surgical microbiology and antibiotic prophylaxis for hair restoration surgery. In: Stough D, Haber R, editors. Hair replacement. St. Louis: Mosby Press; 1996. p. 68–73.

32. Randall JK. Antibiotic use in scalp surgery. In: Unger W, Shapiro R, editors. Hair transplantation. 4th edition. New York: Marcel Dekker, Inc; 2004. p. 2002–4.

33. Farjo N. Infection control and policy development in hair restoration. Hair Transplant Forum International 2008;141–4.

34. Seeery G. Guidelines for designing and location hairlines. Am J Cosm Surg 1998;15(1):21–5.

35. Shapiro R. How to use follicular unit transplantation in the hairline and other appropriate areas. In: Unger W, Shapiro R, editors. Hair transplantation. New York: Marcel Dekker; 2004. p. 454–69.

36. Leavitt M, Perez-Meza D. Technological advances in hair restoration: an examination of the role of the video-microscope. Int J Cosmetic Surg 1998;6(1):76–9.

37. Frechet P. Minimal scars for scalp surgery. Dermatol Surg 2007;33(1):45–55.

38. Perez-Meza D. Factors influencing hair growth and survival. Storage solutions. Multi-chain of reaction. In: Programs and Abstracts. American Academy of Cosmetic Surgery. Jan 2007, Phoenix, AZ.

39. Parsley W. Factors influencing graft survival. Hair Transplant Forum International 2008;126–9.

40. Gandelman M, Mota A, Abrahamsohn P. Light and electron microscopic analysis of controlled injury to follicular unit grafts. Dermatol Surg 2000;26:25–31.

41. Limmer R. Micrograft survival. In: Stough D, Haber R, editors. Hair replacement. St. Louis: Mosby Press; 1996. p. 147–9.

42. Perez-Meza D, Niedbalski R. The use of Custodiol solution for the preservation of hair grafts. In: Programs and Abstracts. 15th Annual ISHRS meeting. Oct 2006. San Diego, CA.

43. Perez-Meza D, Leavitt M, Barusco M. The use of platelet rich plasma for wound healing and as

storage solution during hair transplant surgery. In: Programs and Abstracts. 13th Annual ISHRS meeting. Sidney, Australia 2004.

44. Wasserbauer S, Perez-Meza D, Chao R. Hydrogen peroxide and wound healing: a theorical and practical review for hair transplant surgeons. Dermatol Surg 2008;34(6):745–50.

45. Shiell R. Poor hair growth after hair transplantation: the factor X. In: Stough D, Haber R, editors. Hair transplantation. St. Louis: Mosby; 1996. p. 314–6.

46. Greco JF, Kramer RD. A crush study review of micrograft survival. Dermatol Surg. 1997;23:752–5.

47. Seager D. Micrograft size and subsequent survival. Dermatol Surg 1997;23(9):757–61.

48. Rose P, Parsley W, Perez-Meza D. Skinny Vs chubby grafts. In: program and Abstracts. 8th Annual Orlando Live Surgery Workshop. 2002.

49. Mayer M, Keene S, Perez-Meza D. Graft density production curve with dense packing. In: Programs and Abstracts. 13th Annual ISHRS Meeting. Sydney, Australia. Aug. 2005.

50. Perez-Meza D, Martinick J, Parsley W, et al. Hair graft and survival with sagittal vs coronal recipient sites and dense packing. In: Programs and Abstracts. 14th Annual ISHRS Meeting San Diego, CA. October 2006.

51. Rogliani M, Labardi L, Silvi E, et al. Smokers: risks and complications in abdominal dermolipectomy. Aesthetic Plast Surg 2006;30(4):422–4.

52. Knobloch K, Gohritz A, Reuss E. Nicotine in plastic surgery. Chirug 2008;79(10):956–62.

53. Momeni A, Heier M, Bannash H. Complications in abdominoplasty: a risk factor analysis. J Plastic Reconstr Aesthet Surg 2008; Aug 7 [Epub ahead of print].

54. Ruston Antonio. Tobacco related complications in hair transplant surgery and its treatments. In: Programs and Abstracts. ISHRS Annual meeting 2006. San Diego, CA.

55. Parsley W. Management of the postoperative period: uncommon problems- arteriovenous anastomosis (fistula). In: Unger W, Shapiro R, editors. Hair transplantation. 4th edition. New York: Marcel Decker; 2004. p. 562–3.

56. Weidig JC. Arteriovenous malformation after hair transplantation. In: Stough D, Haber R, editors. Hair replacement. St. Louis: Mosby; 1996. p. 326–7.

57. Davis JS. Scalping accidents. Bulletin Johns Hopkins Hospital 1911;16:259.

58. Coiffman F. Square scalp grafts. Clin Plast Surg 1982;9(2):221–8.

59. Vallis C. Strip scalp graft. Clin Plast Surg 1982;9(2):229–40.

60. Jury J. Use of parieto-occipital flaps in the surgical treatment of baldness. Plast Reconstr Surg 1975;55:456.

61. Ellitot RA. Lateral scalp flap for anterior hairline reconstruction. Clin Plast Surg 1982;9(2):241–53.

62. Alpert B, Buncke H, Mathes S. Surgical treatment of the totally avulsed scalp. Clin Plast Surg 1982;9:145–59.

63. Bell M. Scalp reduction. Clin Plast Surg 1982;9(2):269–78.

64. Leavitt M. Scalp reductions: a modern approach to obtain consistent success. Int J Aest Rest Surg 1995;3(2):95–8.

65. Leavitt M, Perez-Meza D. U-scalp reduction. In: Programs and Abstracts. 3rd Annual Orlando live surgery workshop; 1997.

66. Frechet P. Management of extensive alopecia by scalp extension in combination with occipital slot correction. Int J Aest Rest Surg 1995;3(2):103–14.

67. Frechet P. Scalp extension. In: Unger W, Shapiro R, editors. Hair transplantation. 4th edition. New York: Marcel Dekker, Inc; 2004. p. 765–84.

68. Seery G. Scalp surgery: mechanical and biomechanical considerations. In: Unger W, Shapiro R, editors. Hair transplantation. 4th edition. New York: Marcel Dekker, Inc; 2004. p. 689–97.

69. Marzola M. My approach to alopecia reductions. In: Unger W, Shapiro R, editors. Hair transplantation. 4th edition. New York: Marcel Dekker, Inc; 2004. p. 737–49.

70. Kolasinski J, Kolenda M. Algorithm of hair restoration surgery in children. Plast Reconstr Surg 2003; 112(2):412–22.

How Can Jurors Help Oral and Maxillofacial Surgeons?

W. Scott Johnson, JD*, Gerald C. Canaan II, JD

KEYWORDS

- Oral and maxillofacial surgeons • Patients
- Communication • Litigation • Jurors • Evidence

The United States system of justice, premised on the right to trial by jury, has served all litigants, including oral and maxillofacial surgeons, extremely well since the birth of the nation in 1776. This remarkable system has undergone tremendous change in recent years but not through opinions rendered by courts, nor by changes in statutes made through the legislative process. Instead, the change has taken place in the family rooms of many potential jurors who have become faithful watchers of television shows, such as Crime Scene Investigation (CSI) or Navy Crime Scene Investigation. Informal posttrial interviews of jurors indicate they love the intriguing mystery of determining "who did it." They want empiric evidence, the CSI equivalent of the analysis of a hair or fiber found at the scene of a crime. Jurors enter the courtroom to carry out their civic duties with an expectation that it will take "CSI-type" evidence to prove or defend a case. They want to see the proof. In the last 10 years, the use of audio, video, and PowerPoint evidence at trial has skyrocketed.

WHAT IF THERE IS NO PROVERBIAL "SMOKING GUN"?

Many states have jury instructions that permit the jury to rely on "circumstantial evidence."[a] Another instruction likely tells the jury that they may assign the weight that they choose to give to any evidence. With the "CSI-type" expectations of jurors,

the value of circumstantial evidence and routine practice may take a second chair to the more telling scientific evidence.

To complicate matters, different jurors analyze different evidence in different ways. Some jurors are sensitive, some are jaded, some are flexible, and others are stringent. The list of human qualities is endless as is the bias that jurors bring to the jury box. Patients bring these same biases to a clinician's office during office visits.

Why should one worry about the impact of the "CSI factor" on juries? Are first impressions important? Can anything be learned from these expectations to minimize the risk of civil litigation in oral and maxillofacial surgery cases? The authors submit that it can.

This article presents practical considerations to avoid malpractice claims by approaching the topic through the eyes of a potential juror. Many articles have been written surrounding core risk management practices for oral and maxillofacial surgeons, including appropriate informed consent, surgical preparation, detailed documentation, and appropriate communication.[1] Although articles of this nature are important and a vital part to using good risk management practices, it is also beneficial to approach risk management through the view of those who judge one's actions in court. Using the authors' 30 years of combined experience, this article focuses more on managing the patient by examining the oral and

Hancock, Daniel, Johnson & Nagle, 4701 Cox Road, Suite 400, Glen Allen, VA 23060, USA
* Corresponding author.
E-mail address: sjohnson@hdjn.com (W.S. Johnson).

[a] Circumstantial evidence: 1. Evidence based on inference and not on personal knowledge or observation. — Also termed indirect evidence; oblique evidence. Cf direct evidence (1) 2. All evidence that is not given by testimony. Garner BA, editor in chief. Black's law dictionary. 7th ed. St. Paul, MN: West Group; 1999: 576.

Oral Maxillofacial Surg Clin N Am 21 (2009) 149–153
doi:10.1016/j.coms.2008.10.007
1042-3699/08/$ – see front matter © 2009 Published by Elsevier Inc.

maxillofacial surgeon–patient relationship from the patient's (or potential juror's) viewpoint. Analogies are drawn between the attitudes of jurors and the attitudes of patients.

JURY SELECTION, PATIENT SELECTION

The defense of an oral and maxillofacial surgeon in any jury trial starts with the selection of the jury. The former patient (plaintiff) and his or her attorney sit at one table. The oral and maxillofacial surgeon and his or her attorney occupy another table. Potential members of the jury panel then enter the courtroom. Immediately, before a word is uttered, the attorneys for both the plaintiff and the oral and maxillofacial surgeon begin to process first impressions. What are they wearing? What do they look like? How old are they? What are they carrying with them? Are they dressed appropriately? Are they well groomed? Do they have bad teeth or poor oral hygiene? Is their body language positive or negative? Are they happy or angry? These actions, facial expressions, and appearances create first impressions. Common sense may dictate that potential jurors wearing jeans and a flannel shirt go in one column. Those dressed in a navy blazer and gray dress pants go in another. How about a man with a ponytail or short hair? How about one who is clean shaven? How about one who is reading the *Wall Street Journal* or *People* magazine? Biases, for better or worse, are part of first impressions. For example, one may think that a juror who wears shorts, a t-shirt, and flip flops to court may not care enough about the judicial process to pay attention to the evidence and give the litigants a fair day in court. People who dress "professionally" may or may not be more likely to care. Does the profession of the potential juror make a difference? Do engineers view evidence differently than musicians? Perhaps they do. Does level of education matter? Most lawyers think it does.

That is why attorneys are allowed to ask potential jurors questions through a process called "voir dire."[b] Lawyers love to emphasize how this phrase is enunciated: in the South, it is "voy deer;" in the Southwest, it is "voy dir;" in the North, it is "sit down and answer my questions." In addition to having different pronunciations based on region, voir dire is also handled differently in every state. In some states, voir dire questions are submitted in writing for the jurors to answer, whereas in other states questions are submitted for the trial judge to pose, and still others permit counsel to question potential jurors directly.

The list of questions during jury selection is long and voluminous including in part level of education, work experience, family unit, civic activities, health issues, good or bad experience with oral and maxillofacial surgery or health care, and life experiences that shape their opinions. The voir dire process works only if the attorney takes time to prepare and, more importantly, listen to the answers. Failure to listen may cause valuable information to be ignored, which could jeopardize the defense. Common sense dictates that the attorney for the oral and maxillofacial surgeon should seek out a juror that is conservative, educated, and willing to decide the case on expert testimony and the facts (CSI), not emotions. Is this true? Noted jury consultant Harry J. Plotkin believes that such conclusions are too simplistic.[2]

In Plotkin's opinion, jurors dislike people who are angry, hostile, impatient, condescending, defensive, nervous, hesitant, uncertain, and dishonest.[3] They like people who are professional, honest, courteous, composed, confident, and gracious.[3] Potential patients are looking for the same qualities in an oral and maxillofacial surgeon.

But how can an oral and maxillofacial surgeon convey these subjective character traits to an increasingly objective (CSI) world? Ask the potential patient a lot of questions. Explain exactly what is going to be done, keeping in mind that no two people process information the same way. Indeed, Plotkin[4] opines that there are six different types of personalities in jurors: (1) sympathetic, (2) analytic, (3) practical, (4) conventional, (5) persuasive, and (6) creative.

Sympathetic jurors want to help others. They are caring, nurturing, highly emotional, and feelings-based.[4] The practical juror is the opposite of a sympathetic juror.[5] Practical personalities value pragmatism without emotion.[5] Hard work, common sense, and accomplishment make up their core beliefs.[5] Analytic personalities are calculating, logical, and curious intellects.[6] They enjoy investigations and solving problems.[6] The opposite of an analytic personality is the conventional personality, who views the world in terms of black and white, right and wrong, and in a stark and simplistic way.[7] They do not like complicated analysis.[7] Persuasive personalities are competitive, forceful, and want to be in control of the

---

[b] Voir dire: 1. A preliminary examination of a prospective juror by a judge or lawyer to decide whether the prospect is qualified and suitable to serve on a jury. 2. A preliminary examination to test the competence of a witness or evidence. 3. Hist. An oath administered to a witness requiring that witness to answer truthfully in response to questions. Garner BA, editor in chief. Black's law dictionary. 7th ed. St. Paul, MN: West Group; 1999:1569.

debate.[8] Their goal is to impose their belief on others.[8] Finally, creative jurors are laissez faire, artistic, and open-minded.[9] They are wild cards with an independent streak.[9]

When interviewing and working with patients, surgeons need to consider these six personality traits and take steps to address their varying concerns. Does the patient have a "sympathetic" personality? Make sure he or she knows that the clinician cares about his or her comfort and well-being. When dealing with an analytic patient, be sure to answer the "who," "what," "when," "where," "why," and "how." With creative people, do not confuse their "free spirit" personality with indifference. Make sure they understand exactly what is going to be done. Remember, some patients inherently trust the clinician; others question every move. To determine the personality of the patient, one must ask questions. The equivalent of voir dire in the courtroom setting is the initial assessment and documentation of the patient history. Admittedly, no surgeon enjoys the boring aspects of taking an adequate and detailed history. Instead, surgeons are ready to undertake assessments, make judgments, and determine if they can achieve reasonable expectations. But a rush to surgery without taking adequate time to assess the personality of the patient, question the patient, and listen to the patient can often spell disaster.

Although the written medical history form completed by the patient may be silent, it is incumbent on the surgeon to ask probing questions and listen so that follow-up questions may be asked. Recently, an oral and maxillofacial surgeon called to report a surgical complication. A patient in his early twenties had presented to the surgeon's office and completed a medical history. The surgeon assessed the patient and recommended surgery. The surgical procedure was uneventful and the patient was discharged to the care of his mother. As the surgeon's nurse was assisting the patient into the mother's car, the mother turned and said, "Can I get the doctor's cell phone number? Every time my son has anesthesia for dental surgery, he reacts wildly when the anesthetic wears off at home." That got everyone's attention.

A review of the patient's medical history indicated that the patient had not identified any problems with anesthesia previously. When questioned about this on a follow-up visit the patient said, "You did not ask me if I had problems after surgery. You only asked me if I had a problem during surgery, and I have not had any." As luck would have it, the patient did experience a violent episode within hours after being discharged, which required 9-1-1 emergency services to be dispatched. Fortunately, the patient was transferred to the emergency room where he was discharged after a few hours of observation with no adverse or long-term complications.

When interviewing potential patients, beware of anyone who is not satisfied with the result of prior oral and maxillofacial surgery. To view this in another way, lawyers do not want jurors who have been unhappy with the results of their own oral and maxillofacial surgery (or any surgery for that matter). Why would an oral and maxillofacial surgeon want such a person for a patient? The chance is remote that another oral and maxillofacial surgeon can make the patient happy. For a brief moment a subsequent oral and maxillofacial surgeon may think, "I am different, I am better, I can do this," but common sense needs to prevail and the oral and maxillofacial surgeon should decline the patient. In short, do not allow overconfidence to replace common sense.

JURY EXPECTATIONS, PATIENT EXPECTATIONS

In posttrial interviews, jurors frequently report that the lawyers for both sides are too repetitive. Admittedly, attorneys are trained to elicit testimony at least three times to increase the jury's opportunity to understand that testimony. If a jury is told in the opening statement what the evidence is going to be, and then a witness is called to put on the evidence, and then the jury is told in the closing arguments what the evidence was, the jury should be informed. This system allows lawyers to manage the expectations of the jury. These expectations are first suggested by the lawyer in the opening statement at the beginning of the trial. Lawyers manage the jurors' expectations by telling them what they are going to prove, showing them the proof, and in closing arguments reminding them, "I kept my word. I told you what the evidence would be. I showed it to you. And you should vote to exonerate my client."

Likewise, oral and maxillofacial surgeons must also use the initial assessment to manage patient expectations. An emotionally needy patient who wants to look like a Hollywood actor or actress must be educated about the limits of cosmetic surgery, but one does not know the patient's expectations unless one asks the following: "What are his or her expectations? Where did he or she obtain these expectations? Friends? Other patients? Photos? My Web site?" In all likelihood, the surgeon, too, will tell the patient about the treatment plan, show the patient photos with similar results, and take "before" and "after" photos.

Oral and maxillofacial surgeons also need to question in detail the content of the medical history and find information that may be missing or unintentionally omitted. Pitfalls to avoid are the failure to review a completed medical history, the failure to ask questions about the history, and the failure to document conversations with the patient.

A favorite tactic of attorneys, both plaintiff and defense, is to review the Web site of an oral and maxillofacial surgeon and use portions of it during trial. Plaintiff's attorneys love to compare the "perfect" photos from the Web site with the allegedly imperfect "after" photos of the patient-plaintiff. Surgeons should be cautious if their Web site features glamorous photos, because this could serve as grounds for impeachment or cross-examination. Patients routinely testify at trial that they decided to pursue treatment with the oral and maxillofacial surgeon based on a review of the photos on the surgeon's Web site. The patient, shedding tears, tells the jury that she thought her face would resemble the "Hollywood" faces featured on the Web site.

The surgeon is then called to the stand to testify that as part of the informed consent process, he or she gave the patient numerous disclaimers, minimized expectations, discussed risks, explained potential complications, and did not guarantee any specific outcome. The plaintiff's attorney then shows the jury photos from the oral and maxillofacial surgeon's Web site and asks the oral and maxillofacial surgeon to explain the difference between the glamorous results depicted on the Web site and the suboptimal results that were obtained in the patient. It is hoped that the oral and maxillofacial surgeon can produce a written treatment note that proves that he or she discussed the benefits, risks, alternatives, and expectations with the patient and gave a disclaimer that the photos on the Web site were for illustrative purposes only and results may vary from patient to patient. If the jury can see this treatment note, the oral and maxillofacial surgeon likely wins this issue. Frequently, however, lawyers must defend this issue without the benefit of a detailed note. In that instance, the oral and maxillofacial surgeon normally testifies that he or she "remembers" discussing the issue with the patient because it is their habit to do so. At this point, the oral and maxillofacial surgeon is asking the jury to trust him because there is no direct evidence (CSI) of the discussion. Juries may trust someone they like. The do not trust someone they do not like. When faced with direct CSI-type evidence, however, they view the evidence favorably, even if they do not like the party who benefits from the evidence.

At some point in every trial, the jury must trust an oral and maxillofacial surgeon, but the authors prefer to limit that necessity. This is why they always ask oral and maxillofacial surgeons to remember that when describing events with patients, their memory is rarely available; habits and routines are sometimes available, but good, detailed documentation is always available.

EVIDENCE AT TRIAL, EVIDENCE IN THE OFFICE

Office staff is critical to success. From the receptionists, to the assistants, to the billing coordinators, each person is responsible for ensuring patient safety and satisfaction. Office staff can also, at worst, create liability or, at the least, push an unsatisfied patient toward litigation. Office staff should be an asset, not a liability. But too many times during the litigation process, lawyers have discovered that a patient sued an oral and maxillofacial surgeon client for very subjective reasons: "his receptionist was rude;" "the staff did not respect me;" "the surgeon did not listen to me;" "the office never called me back;" and on and on. These subjective complaints alone are not enough to support a lawsuit against an oral and maxillofacial surgeon, but the negative feelings toward an oral and maxillofacial surgeon invariably push the former patient to visit an attorney's office. When the attorney starts shopping around the surgeon's file, he or she starts piecing together the parts of a malpractice case. Why is office staff important? In most malpractice trials, members of office staff testify, and they are a reflection of the clinician. If jurors think the office staff is mean, rude, disrespectful, or indifferent, then the jurors conclude that the clinician shares those same qualities: "guilty" by association.

How can one rebut allegations from a patient that he or she was treated negatively by office staff? There are two primary methods: hope that most staff members tell the same story to rebut the patient's allegations; and give the jury empiric evidence that proves that the patient's allegations are without merit. Relying on the memory of each staff member is not ideal. Jurors normally discount "memories" of self-serving facts. If office staff have documented their interactions with the patient, however, it can be proved that the patient's allegations are false. Good documentation by staff can also prove that the patient was the rude or disrespectful party. For example, if the scheduling coordinator called the patient to confirm an appointment and the patient responded, "I'll come when I feel like it, you old goat," the time and date of that statement must be recorded in the electronic record or the patient's chart. Clearly, this is an offensive and unwarranted comment that damages the patient's credibility with the jury. But it is much more effective to show the jury (from the documentation) exactly when the statement was made rather than have the scheduler testify, "At some point the patient called me an old goat, but I don't remember when."

How can office staff help the clinician? Encourage everyone to document unusual contact with or comments from patients. Ironically, some oral and maxillofacial surgeons are of the mistaken opinion that nursing and office personnel should not be permitted to document in patient charts. If a patient tells the scheduler or the receptionist anything rude or disrespectful, he or she must document it with objective data. It is not helpful to document that the "patient was angry;" anger is subjective. Instead, the documentation should say, "Patient cussed me out, stated that she will be at our office sometime before noon for her appointment, and hung up on me." Likewise, if a patient sends a complimentary letter, card, or e-mail save it in the chart. The authors have handled several cases where plaintiffs have written letters to clients proclaiming them to be "the greatest oral and maxillofacial surgeons ever" because they restored the patients' oral health. When the patients later sued the clients, the authors showed the jury those letters and watched the plaintiffs squirm in their chairs at trial.

Staff can also help when communicating with patients. Empower staff to report if an entry in the chart is missing. Make sure they know the rules of documentation. Everyone should know that the benefits, risks, and alternatives of the proposed procedure must be documented. The recommendations of the proposed treatment plan must be clear. If the staff does not understand it, neither will the patient. When using electronic records, beware of "one size fits all" entries. Some oral and maxillofacial surgeons use macros that produce the same entry for every problem. Some electronic health record software automatically fills in routine information. This can be a great time saver for the clinician and office staff, but it can be a disaster in court. If jurors see that every patient is given the exact same treatment plan, they conclude that the clinician is not interested in patient care, that they are interested in seeing as many patients as possible to make more money.

There are several ways to make chart entries patient-specific: include the amount of time spent with the patient; document personal details revealed by the patient ("I just returned from vacation"); document anything given to the patient (ie, pamphlet on orthognathic surgery) or anything that the patient may have watched (ie, movie regarding third molar extractions); and document positive comments from the patient ("I love my implants. They restored my confidence."). This type of documentation rebuts allegations to the contrary from the plaintiff and provides the CSI-type proof demanded by today's juries.

SUMMARY

When performing oral and maxillofacial or cosmetic surgery, pretend that the patient is a potential juror who is evaluating one's performance. Determine the personality type of the patient and modify communication style to fulfill that patient's individual needs. Take time to listen. Remember to document both subjective and objective information. Finally, remember that today's jurors (and patients) demand evidence and information that they can see. Blame CSI, but a picture is still worth a thousand words.

REFERENCES

1. Johnson WS. Legal considerations surrounding cosmetic surgery. Oral Maxillofacial Surg Clin N Am 2005;17:123–7.
2. Plotkin HJ. Jury selection. Harry Plotkin Jury Consultant Web Site. Available at: http://www.yournextjury.com. Accessed April 28, 2008.
3. Plotkin HJ. Building trust among the jury: creating positive impressions. Orange County Lawyer 2005; 47(8).
4. Plotkin HJ. Personality types: the sympathetic juror. Harry Plotkin Jury Consultant Web Site. Available at: http://www.yournextjury.com/jt1106.htm. Published November 2006. Accessed April 28, 2008.
5. Plotkin HJ. Personality types: the practical juror. Harry Plotkin Jury Consultant Web Site. Available at: http://www.yournextjury.com/jt1206.htm. Published December 2006. Accessed April 28, 2008.
6. Plotkin HJ. Personality types: the analytical juror. Harry Plotkin Jury Consultant Web Site. Available at: http://www.yournextjury.com/jt0207.htm. Published February 2007. Accessed April 28, 2008.
7. Plotkin HJ. Personality types: the conventional juror. Harry Plotkin Jury Consultant Web Site. Available at: http://www.yournextjury.com/jt0307.htm. Published March 2007. Accessed April 28, 2008.
8. Plotkin HJ. Personality types: the persuasive juror. Harry Plotkin Jury Consultant Web Site. Available at: http://www.yournextjury.com/jt0507.htm. Published May 2007. Accessed April 28, 2008.
9. Plotkin HJ. Personality types: the creative juror. Harry Plotkin Jury Consultant Web Site. Available at: http://www.yournextjury.com/jt0607.htm. Published June 2007. Accessed April 28, 2008.

Index

Note: Page numbers of article titles are in **boldface** type.

A

Ablative laser skin resurfacing, complications of, 9–10
Acne, as complication of skin resurfacing, 4
Allergic reaction, as complication of injectable facial fillers, 21
Allergy, as complication of upper blepharoplasty, 37
Alloplastic augmentation materials, for facial implants, 91–92
Anesthesia, tumescent, for neck liposuction and submentoplasty, 44
Aneurysm, as complication of hair transplant surgery, 145
Antihelical deformities, after otoplasty, 113–115
Arrhythmias, cardiac, as complication from skin resurfacing with deep phenol peels, 7–8
Arteriovenous fistula, as complication of hair transplant surgery, 145
Asymmetry, after placement of facial implants, 102
    as complication of Botox treatment, 16
    as complication of injectable facial fillers, 20
    of eyelid crease after upper blepharoplasty, 34–35
Auditory meatus, external, narrowing of, after otoplasty, 116–117
Augmentation materials, alloplastic, for facial implants, 91–92

B

Bacterial infections, as complication of skin resurfacing, 3–4
Bleeding, as complication of neck liposuction or submentoplasty, 48
    during hair transplant surgery, 122–123
    postoperative, after hair transplant surgery, 135–137
Blepharoplasty, avoiding complications in, **31–41**
    lower eyelid, 37–41
        eyelid malposition, 40–41
    non-sight-threatening complications, 32–34
    patient evaluation checklist prior to, 32–34
    upper eyelid, 34–37
        allergy, 37
        asymmetric eyelid crease, 34–35
        dog ears, 37
        lagophthalmos and dry eye, 37
        medial canthal webbing, 35–36
        milia, 37
        oversculpted deep superior sulcus, 36–37
        skin marking prior to, 34
        wound dehiscence, 37

vision-threatening complications, 31–32
Blood supply, of scalp, in preoperative evaluation for hair transplant surgery, 121
    inadequate, poor results of hair transplant surgery due to, 145
Bone resorption, under facial implants, 101–102
Bony orbits, evaluation of prior to upper blepharoplasty, 32–33
Bony vault, late complications of, after rhinoplasty, 87–88
Botox treatment, complications of, **13–21**
    asymmetry, 16
    bruising, 16–17
    overtreatment, 13–14
    perioral droop, 17
    true eyelid ptosis, 14–15
    undertreatment, 13
    unrealistic patient expectations, 17
Brow lift, nerves at risk for injury during, 25
Brows, evaluation of prior to upper blepharoplasty, 32
Bruising, as complication of Botox treatment, 16–17
    as complication of injectable facial fillers, 18–19
Bulges, as complication of fat grafting, 56

C

Cardiac arrhythmias, as complication from skin resurfacing with deep phenol peels, 7–8
Cartilaginous vault, late complications of, after rhinoplasty, 85–87
Chin implant, nerves at risk for injury during, 25
Communication, avoidance of litigation by considering viewpoint of potential jurors, **149–153**
Complications, of cosmetic surgery procedures, 1–153
    blepharoplasty, **31–41**
    facelift surgery, **59–80**
    facial implants, **91–104**
    facial, nerve injuries in, **23–29**
    fat transfer, **53–58**
    fillers and Botox, **13–21**
    hair restoration surgery, **119–148**
    malpractice claims for. juror and patient viewpoints on, **149–153**
    neck liposuction and submentoplasty, **43–52**
    otoplasty, **105–118**
    rhinoplasty, **81–89**
    skin resurfacing-related, **1–12**
Conchal bowl deformities, after otoplasty, 115
Contact dermatitis, as complication of skin resurfacing, 2–3

Oral Maxillofacial Surg Clin N Am 21 (2009) 155–161
doi:10.1016/S1042-3699(09)00009-0
1042-3699/09/$ – see front matter © 2009 Elsevier Inc. All rights reserved.

Moving?

Make sure your subscription moves with you!

To notify us of your new address, find your **Clinics Account Number** (located on your mailing label above your name), and contact customer service at:

E-mail: elspcs@elsevier.com

800-654-2452 (subscribers in the U.S. & Canada)
314-453-7041 (subscribers outside of the U.S. & Canada)

Fax number: 314-523-5170

Elsevier Periodicals Customer Service
11830 Westline Industrial Drive
St. Louis, MO 63146

*To ensure uninterrupted delivery of your subscription, please notify us at least 4 weeks in advance of move.

Our issues help you manage *yours.*

Every year brings you new clinical challenges.

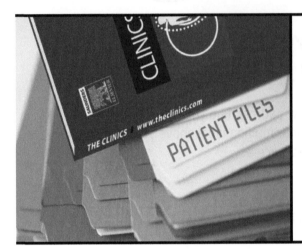

Every **Clinics** issue brings you **today's best thinking** on the challenges you face.

Whether you purchase these issues individually, or order an annual subscription (which includes searchable access to past issues online), the **Clinics** offer you an efficient way to update your know how…one issue at a time.

DISCOVER THE CLINICS IN YOUR SPECIALTY!

Dental Clinics of North America.
Publishes quarterly. ISSN 0011-8532.

Oral and Maxillofacial Surgery Clinics of North America.
Publishes quarterly. ISSN 1042-3699.

Atlas of the Oral and Maxillofacial Surgery Clinics of North America.
Publishes biannually. ISSN 1061-3315.

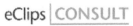

Where the Best Articles become the Best Medicine

Visit **www.eClips.Consult.com** to see what 180 leading physicians have to say about the best articles from over 350 leading medical journals.

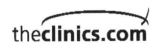

M022487

Printed and bound by CPI Group (UK) Ltd, Croydon, CR0 4YY

03/10/2024

01040361-0016